A Playbook for Weight Loss Success

Sex
ISN'T THE
ONLY WAY
TO HAVE AN
Orgasm

25 Ways to Lose Weight
Through Pleasure

Kristin Heslop, DMA

Flint Hills Publishing

DISCLAIMER:
All information and tools presented within this book are intended for educational purposes. Any health, diet, or exercise advice is not intended as medical diagnosis or treatment. If you think you have any type of medical condition you should, as with all matters, use your own discretion in deciding whether to seek professional advice

Book Design by Thea Rademacher
Author Photograph by Nikki Moore, Nikki Moore Photography
Cover Design by Amy Abrahams:

STONY POINT
Graphics

stonypointgraphics.weebly.com

Flint Hills Publishing

Topeka, Kansas
www.flinthillspublishing.com
Printed in the U.S.A.

ISBN-13:978-0692982464
ISBN-10:0692982469

CONTENTS

~ *A Note to the Reader* ~

This book has been written for you, and it is my hope that you will use it—that you will write in it, make notes in it, mark it up till your heart's content.

When I read a book, I respond to it. I am the type of reader who always reads a book with a pen or pencil in my hand and a highlighter nearby. If I like what a writer has said, I respond with a big "YES" written in the margins. If a writer's words trigger a thought or a memory, I will jot down my ideas in the margin. But if I don't particularly care for what someone has said, I'll just put the book down and walk away. It is my deepest desire that you do not walk away from this book, as this book is for you. This book is for your responses. Please read this book with a pen, pencil, or highlighter nearby.

Each chapter ends with questions that I hope will provoke some thoughts. Please take the time to write down the thoughts that you have, the discoveries that you make, the feelings you feel. I want this to be a book that we write together. And if we do, in fact, write this book together, I have strong intentions and desires around the outcome.

My deepest wish is that you uncover your radiance and discover how fantastic you are. I hope that this book will become a vehicle for you to utterly transform your thinking about your body. I desire that while working together, we will create something that will empower and enliven and help ourselves to discover the women we truly are. And finally, I desire that this book help us squeeze as much pleasure, joy, and delight out of each day as possible.

Kristin Heslop

Preface:
My Weight Loss Story.

I've always hated diets. The only "official" diet I went on was in 1988 when I tried to combine foods. For three days, I combined, and combined, and combined. And promptly got sick.

Thus ended my dieting career.

I'd gained five pounds.

While dieting has never appealed to me, I have been a big fan of binging. I could binge with the best of 'em. I binged on ice cream sandwiches. I binged on entire loaves of homemade bread straight from the oven, with real butter melting into the nooks and crannies. I binged on chocolate covered caramel pecan turtles. I binged on chocolate covered cherries. I binged on croissants. I binged on cinnamon rolls. I binged on Little Debbie Swiss Cake Rolls. I binged on German chocolate cake. I binged on Boston cream pie. I binged on chocolate chip cookies. I binged on chocolate chip cookie dough. I binged on chocolate chips themselves. I binged on only two kinds of pizza, however: hot and cold.

Binging allowed me to numb myself into a psychic oblivion. Although the first bite usually tasted wonderful, at the end of a debauched encounter with an extra-large bag of corn chips and a half-gallon of double chocolate ice cream, I tasted nothing. And I felt nothing, other than post-binge misery, post-binge guilt, post-binge shame, and post-binge frustration.

I was not using food to nourish me.

Instead, I was using food to medicate me—to conceal, deny, repress, and submerge my pain.

During my 20s and 30s, I made two valiant efforts to release weight. These were not diets. These were serious quests to change my lifestyle. During my first attempt, I released 18 pounds, and within a couple of years, I had gained 60. During my second major lifestyle change, I released 40 pounds, and again, within a couple of years, I had regained 30. Each attempt at a healthful lifestyle was short-lived, and each attempt was promptly followed by a weight gain.

These changes were short-lived because I believed that eating less and exercising more was all it took.

I was wrong.

I believed that the only thing I had to do was address the physical things, like food and exercise. I was wrong about that, too. Addressing those issues did not lead to a permanent healthful weight or a permanent sense of well-being. I could temporarily achieve a certain number on the scale, but my biggest problem was that I was ignoring the emotions that were propelling me toward food.

During these years, I criticized and judged myself ruthlessly. I lived in a world of "shoulds." *I should feel happy* or *I shouldn't feel scared* or *I should have drunk more water today* or *I shouldn't have eaten the entire bag of Tostitos.*

And I didn't allow myself to feel negative feelings as they came up. Instead, I ate. A lot.

Two things were missing from my life during those years of binging. First, gratitude. And second, permission. It wasn't until I began to appreciate and be grateful for my body, even with an extra 45 pounds of weight on it, that I began to release the weight. And it wasn't until I permitted myself to feel all of my emotions—the good, the bad, the ugly—that I was able to deal with the negative feelings without being driven to food.

Somebody asked me recently, "What clicked for you?" I wish I could say that it was only one thing that clicked, but actually, it was more of a combination of things. However, the most significant thing I did, and continue to do today, was to consciously and intentionally chose different thoughts about myself and my body. I became hyper-aware of my thoughts about my body and the words I used to describe my body.

Here are a few examples:

> *I'm so fat* became *I'm pretty darn cute.*

> *I can't believe I've allowed this to happen to me—again!—* morphed into *I really love my body!*

> *Ugh! I'm getting my mother's double chin!* became *My hair looks really great today!*

> *I'm so out of shape I can barely walk up the stairs* was transformed into *I have two legs that work really well.*

Which thoughts do you think are more empowering? And which thoughts do you think helped me learn to treat my body with love, compassion, and respect?

It was while I was carrying 45 pounds of unnecessary weight that I began to deeply consider the preciousness of my human body. I decided to view my body with love, rather than disgust and repulsion. I began to notice things about my overweight body that I liked—like my glorious head of hair. Or that I had two legs that have taken me to the tops of mountains and have propelled me through ocean saltwater. Or that my voluptuous, feminine curves could garner masculine attention. Or that every fingernail and toenail was healthy and strong and that each nail protected me as I washed dishes or walked up a flight of stairs.

As I shifted my internal environment from self-loathing to self-love, my external environment began to shift as well. I began to consider the question, "What will bring me the most pleasure?" And the answer to that question usually had to do with sustaining myself with nourishing food, honoring my body with rest and movement, and feeding my mind and spirit with nourishing thoughts. Suddenly, fresh pineapple and strawberries brought me more pleasure than french fries, and taking a little walk around the block was more pleasurable than coffee and a candy bar.

If binging is a part of your life, as it was a part of my life for so many years, please consider two things. First—notice, approve of, and embrace all of your feelings—even the ugly ones, the unpleasant ones, and the ones you wish would go away. And second, every time you glimpse yourself in the mirror, say, "I'm pretty darn cute."

1: What Will Bring You the Most Pleasure?

Human beings, by changing the inner attitudes of their minds, can change the outer aspects of their lives.

~ William James

Everywhere we look, we see women—women who are maybe unhappy, depressed, or just a little sad. Perhaps these women feel empty or powerless or stressed. Maybe they're in pain. Maybe they feel numb or fatigued. If you were to ask these same women to talk about their bodies, I can almost guarantee you that they'd be able to list 100 things about their bodies that make them unhappy: *My ass is too fat. My breasts are too big. My breasts are too small. My hair is too gray. My hair is too curly. My hair is too frizzy. My pores are too big. That zit is ugly. My thighs have so much cellulite. My stomach is fat. I have noodle arms. I'm too old. I'm too fat.*

And here's something else about women: we're killing ourselves. The hatred we hold in our hearts toward our physical bodies is, perhaps, a slow form of suicide. As we devalue our bodies, we die a slow, emotional death. Perhaps we are too busy, too stressed, too overbooked. Perhaps we don't have enough time to spend with our families, or to spend alone with ourselves. Perhaps we are eating on the run, eating from vending machines in the break room, eating meal after meal at convenience stores or gas stations. Is this causing our slow death?

Maybe.

Perhaps we are putting everyone else's "needs" ahead of ourselves while ignoring our fundamental need for pleasure.

What happens to us as adults when we receive no pleasure?

We die.

We die by attempting to find pleasure in places that really can't provide true satisfaction. We die when we put other's needs ahead of our own and at the same time, we die when we expect that these people will be able to read our minds and know what we need without our asking for it. Occasionally, or maybe frequently, we expect that others in our lives will be able to magically intuit our deepest desires. This can create an interesting phenomenon—we want other people to make us happy. We want others to create for us a pleasure-filled life. We expect other people to make us happy when we ourselves can't even identify what would make us happy. We think that by serving others and taking care of others, those same people will read our minds and our hearts and will magically eventually reciprocate in exactly the way we want them to.

But that will never happen.

When we give others the responsibility for making us happy, they may fail at the job, and then we feel pissed. And rather than dealing with the negative feelings as we're having them, in an honest and forthright way, it becomes really easy for us to repress, deny, medicate, and numb ourselves with a Snickers bar and a Coke.

If you are reading this book, then like me, you have faced very personal issues regarding your relationship with your body. You have faced challenges with your decisions about food.

I've been exactly where you are.

And through a lot of deep soul-searching, I've found a new paradigm about my body and food that has positively changed my life.

I'm asking you to trust me, to explore in your own mind and heart, my discoveries.

As we'll delve into more deeply throughout this book, there is a fundamental concept you must understand in order to bring about a shift in your relationship with your body:

The key to beginning the shift is to ask yourself:

What will bring me the most pleasure?

It is up to each of us, as women, to figure out what will bring us pleasure, the most pleasure, and then make sure that we get that. If eating a Snickers bar from the vending machine will bring you pleasure, eat it. If you'd rather be pleasured by exquisite dark chocolate from Godiva, eat that. If you can honestly say that fast food will pleasure you, eat fast food!

But while fast food might bring you some sort of short-lived, temporary pleasure, will it bring you the *most* pleasure? Will french fries *really* lead you to your body's desires? Will Ben and Jerry guide you on the path to rapturous body love? Probably not.

Maybe for you, the most pleasure might come from taking your own sweet time in the produce section of the grocery store: buying a whole pineapple, taking delight in the process of selecting the perfect fruit, the perfect size, enjoying bringing it home, putting it on the dining room table as a centerpiece to let it ripen a little more, enjoying its look, shape, texture, and color, relishing the sound of the knife as you cut through its spiny skin, slurping the juice that spills from its flesh as you slice it up, taking pleasure in the tangy sweetness as you chew it, and then feeling great that you just did something wonderful for your body. Perhaps that large order of fries won't give you the most pleasure. Perhaps indulging in the pleasure of pineapple will.

"But I'm too busy. I have kids, a husband, a house to look after, my elderly mother, and a full-time job! Everybody's depending on me! I'm too busy taking care of others. Who has time for pleasure?" I hear you say. You have all sorts of demands on your time. You barely have time to cruise through the drive-thru, much less take time to "prioritize your pleasure." Well, what you don't deal with now, you *will* eventually deal with. If you don't deal with your pleasure now (taking care of your body, asking your body what it wants), you will be forced to deal with it, either in the form of diabetes, high blood pressure, osteoporosis, arthritis, cancer, heart attack, stroke, various joint replacements. Your body may be crying out to you, "Love me now. Love me now!" but because you're "too busy," you're ignoring it. Like a little child who cries until it is fed, or a pet who whines until you take it out, your body *will* find a way to get its needs met. And wouldn't it be much more pleasurable to listen to its needs now, voluntarily, before it cries loudly for your attention later?

The reason I'm aware of what women say and how these women behave and what women look like and what women do—is because I am a woman. I spent the first 44 or so years of my life in self-loathing, hating my body, despising everything about my body, and perhaps even wishing that I didn't inhabit my body. I was too fat, too clumsy, too out of shape, my breasts were too big, my ass was too big, my stomach was too big, I was too big. The list went on and on. I hated looking at myself in the mirror. I hated catching glimpses of my reflection in storefront windows. I hated seeing myself in pictures.

But I am happy to report that you don't have to remain trapped within the quagmire of regretful thoughts and painful feelings. There is another way. It's a path toward self-love. It is possible to move from self-loathing to self-appreciation.

There's a process to this, and I want to show you how you create a cherished, long-term, loving relationship with your body—and yourself—as well.

In my heart, I know that my relationship with my body is the most important thing I'm here to learn. How I feel about my body, how I relate to my body, has—and continues to be—the major theme in my life.

So it bears repeating. . . the most important question you can ask yourself is:

What will bring *me* the most pleasure?

When you're in doubt, when you feel confused, stressed out, upset, bored, or angry, ask yourself this. Your answer will prioritize things. It will put situations into focus. It will bring clarity to your viewpoint and things will crystallize.

Though it may seem like an easy question, if you've never deeply contemplated what will truly give you the most pleasure, you may find it difficult to get started thinking about the answer. Delve into the following exercise and you may discover that your body is giving you some serious information on the subject of pleasure.

How to Listen to Your Body.

Easier said than done, right? Indeed, our bodies are always talking to us. But how often do we really pay attention to what they're saying?

My biggest challenges occur when I ignore the messages my body sends me. Here are a few things that my body says to me from time to time:

"Move me!"

"Let me rest!"

"Give me peace!"

"Give me action!"

"Feed me."

"Stop feeding me!"

"Stretch me!"

"Ice me!"

"Massage me!"

I find that the more I listen to my body, and the more I do what she says, the happier I am, the more energy I have, and the better I feel. So, if you feel disconnected from your body, here are a few tips to establish a fantastic connection to her.

TIP ONE: Master the Fine Art of Curiosity.

I began my weight-release journey basically out of curiosity. I began to think, *I wonder what would happen if I got in the best shape of my life. I wonder how I would feel if I started eating really, really well. I wonder what would happen if I really figured out this exercise thing. I wonder what would happen if I started saying loving, compassionate things to myself."* And as I became curious about "what would happen if. . ." my body responded to my curiosity in miraculous ways.

TIP TWO: Master the Fine Art of Appreciation.

Recently, after a day of strenuous physical activity, I thanked my body with a warm soak—in delightfully warm water, Epsom salts, and lavender oil. As I was soaking in a tub full of warm water, I poked, prodded, dug around in, and massaged my calf muscles vigorously. And while I massaged them, I thanked them for carrying me throughout the day. I thanked them for being strong and healthy for the past several months. And I thanked them for allowing me to experience the simple pleasure of movement.

TIP THREE: Ask Your Body What She Wants.

Sit quietly. Take a few deep breaths, and in your mind, ask your body what she wants. Listen for the response. She will always tell you if you ask her. Does she want more rest? Does she want to eat more healthful food? Does she want to be outdoors more? Does she want more time alone? What does your body really, really want?

Be curious about your body.

Appreciate your body.

Ask her to talk to you and when she talks, listen!

Listen to your body. Listen to your heart. And then do what your body and heart are asking you to do.

Record what your body tells you she wants:

_____

_____

_____

_____

_____

_____

_____

_____

_____

_____

_____

_____

Kristin Heslop

Playtime: Examine Your Happiness.

Take a moment, light a candle, make some tea or coffee or pour yourself a glass of wine, put on some music, sit down, breathe, and start to answer these questions:

What makes you happy?

Remember, diets help us gain wait. Pleasure helps us release weight because we trust what our bodies are telling us. I want you to contemplate **joy**.

When have you been the happiest? Where were you? What were you doing? What were you seeing? What were you smelling? What were you hearing? What were you tasting? What were you feeling? Were you with people? Were you alone?

Think about your joy, your pleasure, your delight. Get it clear in your mind then put pen to paper and write down your thoughts about when you have felt the most pleasure. Investigate your happiness, your pleasure, your joy, your satisfaction, your contentment. Want *extra credit*? Examine your bliss and your ecstasy.

_____

_____

_____

_____

_____

_____

_____

_____

_____

_____

_____

_____

_____

Kristin Heslop

_____
_____
_____
_____
_____
_____
_____
_____
_____
_____
_____
_____
_____
_____
_____
_____
_____
_____
_____
_____
_____
_____
_____
_____
_____
_____
_____
_____
_____
_____
_____
_____
_____
_____

2. Fall in Love with Your Body.

To love deeply in one direction makes us more loving in all others.
~ Anne-Sophie Swetchine, *The Writings of Madame Swetchine*

What do we mean when we use the term *fall in love*?

What happens when we fall in love? We focus our energy on our beloved. Our lover is continually present in our minds and our cells throb with excitement in anticipation of being together. We revel in every minute we spend with each other. We are open, interested, and curious about everything related to the object of our desire—their past, present, and future. We adore and accept and approve of each other. We complement, praise, and acknowledge each other. We shower each other with affection and warmth. We take pleasure in making each other happy, in making each other smile. We laugh, tease, giggle, and play. We spend lots of time together. We listen. We appreciate everything about our beloved. And on a deeper level, we accept every part of our beloved—their humanness and flaws and frailties, as well as their strengths. We are open to all of them. We connect with each other deeply, intimately, and spiritually. We feel compelled to merge with them, to inhale and be inhaled by them, to devour and be devoured by them. What makes our beloved happy makes us happy.

Now, how would our lives and our bodies change if we treated ourselves like we treat a new love?

Would we lavish ourselves with the attention and love and energy we give to our beloved? If we can't give it to ourselves, who can? How can anyone else love our bodies if we aren't able to?

You've probably heard the following phrase many times, and there is good reason for that as it contains a profound wisdom:

Before you can love others, you must learn to love yourself.

If we do not feel love for ourselves, we will not understand the nature of love and won't be able to share a healthy, balanced love with others. This understanding uncovers even more fundamental truths:

Ultimately, we are personally responsible for our own pleasure and our own happiness.

Ultimately, we are responsible for what we put in our mouth.

Ultimately, we are responsible for loving ourselves and for loving our bodies!

Sadly, women are not given the space, the opportunity, or the language to celebrate themselves. Consequently, it becomes easier to bond through complaining. And when we complain, very often we complain about our bodies, which is harmful. The sad thing is that as we complain about our bodies, we're complaining about our souls.

Wouldn't it be wonderful if we could celebrate every inch of ourselves? Wouldn't it be fantastic if we could enjoy, relish, and take great pleasure in every inch of ourselves, rather than demean our bodies? And if we could verbally appreciate and approve of our bodies, if we could take pleasure in them, then maybe we could find a way to be kinder to them. Maybe we could find a way to listen to our bodies before they resort to drastic means to demand attention. Maybe we could learn to listen to what our bodies are saying to us about the food we feed them, the activities we take part in, and what we say to them and about them.

Wouldn't it be wonderful if we could celebrate our bodies easily?

Perhaps you feel a hesitation to fully embrace this concept. Maybe you have concerns that the whole idea of falling in love with one's body might seem egotistical. Maybe it feels vain and narcissistic. But is it?

Absolutely not.

It's the opposite.

Falling in love with your body is about uncovering and discovering truth.

Falling in love with your body is not about being selfish. Falling in love with your body is not about being inconsiderate or insensitive to other people. Falling in love with your body means that because you adore your body and appreciate your gorgeous physical self, you feel good. And when you feel good, those feelings radiate and spread to others. Loving your body is actually a way to love others in your environment, as well as to take responsibility for your happiness and pleasure. It is a way to guarantee that you understand yourself and that you don't feel angry that someone else isn't making you happy. Loving your body guarantees that you will find pleasure, regardless of your circumstances. When your light is turned on, it blesses the world and allows others to shine as well. But the way to turn on that light, and to bring joy, radiance, and beauty into your world, is to fall in love with your body right here, right now, regardless of the shape, or the size, or the number on the scale. If you're alive, then regardless of your current physical condition, you have something to love.

"Love your neighbor as yourself," Jesus said. And so sprung up an entire religious and ethical system based on "loving your neighbor," or theoretically at least. But sadly, who is teaching us to observe the "as yourself" part? Who is teaching us how to love ourselves? Does the media? Do we learn to love ourselves through on-the-job training? Do public schools off courses in self-love? No.

Perhaps the key word in this concept is love. Dr. Bernie S. Siegel, in *Love, Medicine, and Miracles*, writes, "The ability to love oneself, combined with the ability to love life, fully accepting that it won't last forever, enables one to improve the quality of their life."

Women can certainly release unnecessary weight based on a deep feeling and sense of love—a love of themselves, a love of beautifully prepared, nutritious food, a love of movement—and, maybe, at a deep level, our love for our bodies is spiritual work. Connecting love to our physicality—our hands, our hair, our noses, our toes, our knees, our butts, our spines, or our brains—connecting the love essence to ourselves can and does shift everything.

What would happen if we were to love our bodies?

Perhaps we would treat our bodies with care.

Perhaps we might pay attention to our bodies.

We might listen to our bodies carefully.

We might honor our bodies' needs.

When our bodies are tired, we might let them sleep.

And when our bodies are hungry, we might feed them what they are truly hungry for
(which may or may not be fast food).

The Case for Loving Your Body When You're Really Thinking,
"Why Bother? I'm Too Far Gone."

What's the point of all this? Why should I even bother? Does it even matter? Is it even worth the effort? Perhaps the underlying question is, "Am I even worth the effort?"

Here are a few reasons that might convince you that it is worth the effort—that *you* are worth the effort.

- You might choose to love your body because it's more fun than loathing your body.

- You might choose to love your body because you have it, and it's yours.

- You might choose to love your body because you'll feel better about yourself if you do.

- You might choose to love your body, because it's really good for both your physical and mental health.

- You might choose to love your body because, if you're able to read this, your body has served you in many ways.

- You might choose to love your body because the energy you generate in doing so will not be separated from your environment. It will spread into your environment.

- You might choose to love your body because doing so will give you more energy.

- You might choose to love your body because it's the only one you have.

- You might choose to love your body because when you do, you will probably improve its care and feeding a little bit.

- You might choose to love your body because it's talking to you right now, but are you listening?

- You might choose to love your body because it will improve your health: the way you perceive yourself has a direct correlation with your physiological functioning.

- You might choose to love your body because if you don't love it, nobody else will—except you don't really want to love it to get somebody else to love it, although that may be a happy by-product.

- You might choose to love your body because it deserves to be loved and it has served you well.

So why do I love my body? Because it gives me great orgasms, with or without a partner. I love my body because even when I wasn't there for it, it was there for me. I love my body because it is free of cancer, when for a period of about three weeks, I thought cancer might have made itself a home in my breast. I love my body because it allows me to lay stretched out on my couch, wrapped in blankets and cats and it allows my hand to move across the page to convey my thoughts. I love my body because of the almost orgasmic high I feel after a great run. I love my body because my body is responsive. It adapts and molds itself to my thoughts: if I think I'm fat, I gain weight. If I think I'm slender, I release weight. I love my body because it is flexible and adaptable and malleable. I love my body because it supports me. I love my body because its cyclic nature puts me in touch with the cyclic nature of the earth. I love my body because it's not boring and static, it's always changing, always moving, always in a state of flux, always ebbing and flowing, never staying the same.

Playtime: Now It's Your Turn.

What aspects of your body do you love? How have they served you? How have you shown them that you love them? Write a paragraph about why you love (or should love!) your body:

_____

_____

_____

_____

_____

_____

_____

_____

_____

_____

_____

_____

_____

_____

_____

_____

_____

_____

_____

_____

_____

_____

_____

_____

_____

_____

_____

_____

Next, write the story of your relationship with your body.

How did you feel about your body when you were little?

What were the events that occurred as you grew that impacted your relationship with your body?

What did you like to do as a little child? Sandbox? Freeze tag? Four square? How has your relationship with your body changed over the years? Did something happen? Did someone comment?

What is your body's story?

If your body could talk, what would it say?

Extra credit: What would you say back to your body? How would you respond to it?

_____

_____

_____

_____

_____

_____

_____

_____

_____

_____

_____

_____

_____

_____

_____

_____

_____

_____

_____

3: Why Diets Don't Work and Why Pleasure Does.

Yes, it's true that the senses can lead you astray, and the pursuit of pleasure can get you in trouble. Sensual pleasure needs the guidance of practical and ethical judgment. But you won't gain good health by repeatedly vetoing the vote of the senses and denigrating the wisdom of the body. Nature was not capricious nor perverted in making sure that, other things being equal, what feels good is good for you.

~ George Leonard

Why do diets fail? And why does pleasure work? Look at the first three letters in the word "diet."

They spell "die."

And that's what happens.

When we're on a diet, what do we want to do? We want to die! Why? Because we're depriving ourselves and our bodies. Because we're hungry. Because a diet gives us a list of foods we can eat and we can't eat. Then, after a few days on the diet, we start to feel stressed, angry, tired, or bored! We immediately choose the foods from the list we can't have. And then we feel bad and guilty and that makes us want to eat more of those very foods we can't have.

You can't sustain something that isn't fun. If you feel miserable while you're doing it, why would you keep doing it? If something hurts you or causes you pain, you stop doing it. If your needs aren't being met (like you're not eating enough on the latest crash diet), you will find a way to meet those needs. And off the diet you'll go.

The diet industry and the weight loss industry will fail you every time. Diets force you to follow a faulty premise. That premise is: "I feel bad about myself so I will deprive myself of foods I love. Then, as the days go by, I'll feel worse. I'll go off my diet. Then I'll feel even worse. In frustration (and gnawing hunger) I'll give up, regain weight, and put myself back at square one, which is feeling bad. And then I'll go on another diet!"

It's in the best interest of the diet industry that you continue to feel bad, because your unhappiness is a great motivator. Your unhappiness motivates you to continue to search for the perfect diet, the diet you think you will succeed at following this time. You believe that the latest diet will be the cure all, the panacea, the miracle you've been longing for. You hope that the latest diet will instantly give you the body of your dreams. But a diet will fail you every time. Diets simply perpetuate the vicious circle of grasping at something outside of yourself (a diet, a weight-loss promise, and false hope) to make you happy. And I'm here to say that something outside of yourself will never make you happy.

The only thing that can make you happy is you!

Strict adherence to a diet will never make you happy. A number on a scale certainly can't make you happy. But what does make you happy? Pleasure. Feeling good. And knowing that you are in charge of your pleasure, your good feelings, your fun, and your happiness.

Depriving yourself of foods that you enjoy doesn't bring you pleasure. Restricting yourself and making yourself suffer doesn't bring you pleasure. So, we're back to the most important question you can ask yourself: "What will bring me the most pleasure?"

Playtime: What Will Bring You the Most Pleasure?

Review the Happiness List from Chapter 1 (page 15) that you compiled. Do one of those items on the list and then write about it.

_____

_____

_____

_____

_____

_____

4. The Great Desires List.

Your desire is your prayer. Picture the fulfillment of your desire now and feel its reality, and you will experience the joy of the answered prayer.

~ Dr. Joseph Murphy

What do you really want for your body?

How do you feel about your body right now?

What are the deepest desires you have for your body?

Do you want more energy? Maybe you want to release some extra pounds? Do you want to be able to walk up a flight of stairs and not feel winded? Perhaps your desire is to be able to walk out to your mailbox and not feel out of breath? Do you want to be able to cross your legs easily? Or bend over to tie your shoes without having to sit down? Maybe you want to lower your blood pressure, or reduce certain medications? Or avoid certain medications altogether?

Ask yourself, "What do I *really* want for my body?"

Attend to your answers with honesty and truth, and write them down here:

_____

_____

_____

_____

_____

_____

_____

_____

_____

_____

_____

_____

_____

_____

_____

_____

_____

_____

_____

_____

_____

_____

_____

_____

_____

_____

_____

_____

_____

_____

_____

_____

_____

_____

_____

_____

_____

_____

_____

_____

_____

Now, think about how great you will feel when these desires all come to fruition. Think about how wonderful and proud you'll feel when you release the pounds, or when your doctor takes you off the meds, or when you feel filled with exuberance and vitality and energy. Visualize it. Imagine it. Rehearse it in your mind. See yourself inhabiting the body you desire.

Here is my personal experience with the power of desire. I have had phenomenal success in releasing unnecessary weight, and also success in maintaining its release. Here is what I did. And you can do it, too. It's easy! And oh-so-pleasurable! The biggest part is asking yourself, "What do I want? What do I desire?"

A few years ago, some friends and I decided to meet regularly and talk about our desires. At the beginning of that month, I made an extravagantly long list of desires, many pertaining to my body. I felt that that year would be a great year to begin a new project. The project of my choice? A fantastic relationship with my body. For a while, I had heard ideas floating around to the effect that, *if you want to change the world, change yourself. Be the change you wish to see in the world.* I knew that the change I wanted to create in the world was a new body—a healthy, fit, and beautiful body. Here are my desires as I embarked on my weight release journey:

I desire a smokin' hot body.

I desire a firm, muscular, beautiful body.

I desire to infuse pleasure and fun into physical fitness.

I desire to get physically fit.

I desire to have my outside reflect my inside—I've done so much work on my heart and my head that I'm ready for my body to reflect the beauty that is in my soul.

I desire to get in the peak physical condition of my life!

I desire to find a way to enjoy getting in peak physical condition.

I desire to say loving, positive things to myself about my body and about working out.

I desire that my body weight is in my ideal weight range.

I desire to be a size 12.

I desire a toned and defined body.

I desire a voluptuous, curvy, shapely, and healthy body.

I desire lots and lots of endurance.

I desire lots of flexibility.

I desire lots of strength.

I desire to continue to look at my body and say positive things about my body and to appreciate my physical appearance.

I desire to look great in shorts.

I desire to say loving, understanding, compassionate words to myself.

I desire to enjoy moving my body.

We all know the principles of reducing weight. It's not rocket science. In fact, it's really just common sense. Eat lots of fruits and vegetables. Drink a lot of water. Move more. Keep a food journal. Eat sensible portions. No big surprise here. Any magazine, diet book, or weight loss program will tell you the same thing. For me, and probably for most people, knowing what to do isn't the problem. I have "known" what to do all of my life. The problem comes in the "doing" part. For me, the best way to "do it" would be through the power of my desires and the power of pleasure.

Playtime: The Great Desires List.

What do you want? Give yourself a little bit of space and time to relax and think and breathe and then jot down every single desire you have for your body. What do you want? How do you want to feel? What do you want to do? Are there health outcomes you're looking for? Write them down. Is there a clothing size that you're considering? Write it down. Is there a number on the scale? Write it down. Do you want more energy? Do you want less fatigue? Do you want to simply feel better about yourself? Be as specific as you can be.

Write it down, in glorious detail:

_____

_____

_____

_____

_____

_____

_____

_____

_____

_____

_____

_____

_____

_____

_____

_____

_____

_____

_____

_____

Kristin Heslop

5. Put the Pleasure Back in Eating.

Man is not free to refuse to do the thing which gives him more pleasure than any other conceivable action.

~ Stendhall

Fast, fast, fast!

Go, go, go!

Now, now, now!

We want what we want. We want it now. We become frustrated when things don't happen quickly enough to make us happy. And it seems that this desire for speed in our lives impacts the way we eat.

We eat on the run. We eat on the go. We eat on the job. We eat in the car. We eat while we're doing other things. We eat while we're working, watching TV, at the movies. We even eat while we're shopping for food, thanks to the handy little round beverage container attached to the grocery cart we're pushing. "Drink it now, and pay later," it suggests. We can rest assured that we will certainly be paying for that soft drink, not only with our wallet, but with our health and our bodies as well.

How many times have we had a stressful day at work? On the way home, we stop by the gas station to fill up our cars with the cheapest gas we can find. While gassing up the car, we notice a two-for-one special on chips, and a buy-one-get-one-half-price special on pop, and our favorite candy is on sale, too! We get home, turn on the TV, sit down in our recliner with the remote, and open the bag of chips.

As we're watching the latest reality show, we begin to put food in our mouth—mindlessly. Before you know it, we've polished off both bags of chips, the soda, and the candy. But we've tasted none of it. We put the food in our mouth, chewed it up, and swallowed it, but we were blissfully unaware of any of it. We weren't enjoying it. We were relishing it. We weren't tasting it at all.

Is there a correlation between overeating and mindless eating? While we're eating mindlessly, we're unaware of what we're putting in our mouths. We certainly are not paying attention to what we're eating, how much we're eating, and how we're feeling as we're eating. Eating mindlessly can easily lead to eating copious quantities of food and not even being aware that it's happened.

But the good news is, mindless eating can be cured with sensual eating! Try thinking pleasurable, sensual thoughts about the food that is in front of you. Really look at what it is you're eating. Enjoy the color, the appearance, the aroma. Take pleasure in the texture and taste. Really feel the food on your lips and tongue, and enjoy all of it by being hyper-aware as you're eating it.

It is so important that what we eat, what we put in our mouths, pleases us, and that we're eating to bring ourselves pleasure. This idea, which I believe is fundamental to long-term success, runs counter to the general perception that to lose weight, you must eat certain foods regardless of your personal preferences. Therefore, another critical factor in infusing pleasure into your weight release efforts is to only eat foods you like. Never eat foods you don't like. Not a fan of carrots? Don't eat them. Not crazy about spinach? Just say no! You've had it up to here with iceburg lettuce? That's fine, too. Just leave it alone! Only eat foods that you love.

This concept may strike you as exactly the opposite of what you've come to understand.
Typically, when we try to lose weight, we put ourselves on a diet, and an inherent part of that plan is that we restrict our food choices.

This way of thinking contradicts a fundamental way our brain works. When we were hunters and gatherers, during a meal our brains would say to us, "Eat! Eat! Eat! You have no idea when you'll find food again!" In effect, our brains evolved in a way that rejected willpower. Modern scientific research confirms this idea. In general, if you deprive yourself of something, like attention, affection, or particular foods, your brain will just want it more! So, once you come off a restrictive diet, you may be *more* likely to binge.

We need to realize that telling our brains "no" in a significantly-restricted way, and then expecting to have long-term healthy habits, is a recipe for failure.

If you deprive yourself of what you truly enjoy, what will happen when you get home at 6 o'clock on a Friday night, after a long week at work? What will happen when you come home, tired and hungry? If you're like most people, there's a pretty good chance that you'll end up eating a whole lot of what you've not allowed yourself to eat.

Geneen Roth in *When You Eat at the Refrigerator, Pull Up a Chair*, suggests that you carry a piece of chocolate with you everywhere you go. What a pleasurable idea! Give yourself the freedom and permission to eat what you want, when you want it. Sometimes just knowing that you could have it, if you really want it, is enough. You don't even have to eat it. Just knowing that you have the option may be enough. And you might ask yourself, *Do I really want that piece of chocolate? Or would an apple and a granola bar be more filling, more satisfying, and bring me deeper pleasure? Or maybe I'm just thirsty for a tall, refreshing glass of water? Or would I be happier having a big, delicious, fresh salad?*

Again, we're back to the question of "What would bring you the *most* pleasure?"

In discovering ways to fall in love with your body, that is the one critical, crucial, fundamental, and integral question to ask: What would bring you the most pleasure? When your answer to that question is clear, look at that food. Smell it. Touch it. Taste it. And relish every moment of it.

Playtime: Bring Your Favorite Restaurant Home.

When do you eat mindlessly? Is it in the car? After work? At work? At the end of the day? In front of the television? After experiencing stress? Or joy? Or celebration? Or when you're with others? Or when you're alone? Take note of your mindless eating situations and jot them down here:

_____
_____
_____
_____
_____
_____
_____
_____
_____
_____
_____
_____
_____
_____
_____
_____
_____
_____
_____
_____

_____
_____
_____
_____
_____
_____
_____
_____
_____
_____
_____
_____
_____
_____
_____
_____
_____
_____
_____
_____
_____
_____
_____
_____
_____
_____
_____
_____
_____
_____
_____
_____
_____

How can you infuse pleasure into your food intake? Think about your favorite restaurant. What do you like about it? Is it just the food? Or is it more than the food? Is it the atmosphere, the lighting, the place setting, the music, the candles, the flowers, the décor? What can you do to infuse sensory pleasure into your intake of nourishment?

_____

_____

_____

_____

_____

_____

_____

_____

_____

_____

_____

_____

_____

_____

_____

_____

_____

_____

_____

_____

_____

_____

_____

_____

_____

6. Good Morning, Hot Stuff! I Hope You Live Forever!

Love your neighbor as yourself.

You've heard the Golden Rule?

"Do unto others as you would have them do unto you."

And you've probably heard the second part of it, too: "Love your neighbor as you love yourself."

The message behind these two ideas is simple—be kind to others. Churches, charities, religious teachers and preachers succeed magnificently in telling us to be nice to others. But what is almost universally neglected is the second part of the statement: "Love your neighbor *as you love yourself.*"

Most of us do a pretty good job at loving other people, at loving our neighbors. As women, we're skilled at supporting, praising, encouraging, uplifting, and putting our attention on other people. We're trained at a very early age to nurture and take care of others.

But who teaches us to love ourselves? Who teaches us to lavish ourselves with the loving attention that we put on others in our lives? No one. Is this rooted in the idea, perhaps a misguided fear, that "loving ourselves" would push us toward narcissism and arrogance? Rhonda Byrne writes in *The Secret,* "Many of us were taught to put ourselves last, and as a consequence, we attracted feelings of being unworthy and undeserving. As those feelings lodged within us, we continued to attract more life situations that had us feel more unworthy and not enough. You must change that thinking."

In an effort to avoid egocentrism, I have witnessed many women move in the direction of self-denigration. We use words and language to do anything but express love for ourselves. We are not given the techniques, tools, or words to use to love our bodies and to love ourselves. Was there a course in any of my academic training that taught me how to love myself and my body? No. Did I learn how to love myself in any of my on-the-job training? No.

So, the question is; how can we learn to love ourselves and our bodies if we are given no support, encouragement, or education in this regard? How can we learn to appreciate our physical selves?

Here's how. . .

First, become hyper-aware of the thoughts and the words you use to describe your body. Positive self-talk is a fundamental, crucial, critical aspect in learning how to fall in love with your body. What you say to yourself, internally, mentally, has huge ramifications for the rest of your life because you're impressing your subconscious. Your outside reflects your inside. Your physical self is a mere reflection of the thoughts you have been thinking. Now, if you're thrilled by the body you've created for yourself, you're probably not reading this book. But if you are less than thrilled, and you would like to learn how to love your body, then pay attention to the words you use when you talk to yourself. Starting now.

When you look at yourself in the mirror, what do you say? "I'm ugly?" "I'm fat?" "I hate my body?" Those words have to be eliminated now, now, now, from your vocabulary. You must replace them with positive words like, "I'm adorable," "I'm luscious," "I'm exquisite." You may not want to hear this. You may rebel against this. You may resist this. You may think this is silly, superficial, and stupid. "I'm not adorable," you may say. "I'm not luscious," you may think. "I am so the opposite of exquisite," you may observe.

"Do I really have to say all these nice things to myself?" And to that, I say, "Yes, yes, and yes." Sure, at the beginning, you may think this is stupid. But what I'm asking you to do is unlearn years of negative self-talk that has become so ingrained in your thinking, feeling, and being. How many negative things have you told yourself, about yourself, over the years? And these are not helpful thoughts. They're not uplifting. They don't do anything for anyone, least of all you. All they do is make you feel tired, low, sad, depressed, and maybe a little hopeless.

Playtime: Body Thoughts.

Take a moment and make a list of every thought you think about your body. What do you think about your face, hair, eyes, mouth, nose, cheeks, neck, shoulders, back, arms, hands, belly, butt, thighs, knees, calves, ankles, feet—you get the picture.

Put a timer on for one minute. Write it down. Write it down fast:

_____

_____

_____

_____

_____

_____

_____

_____

_____

_____

_____

_____

_____

Now, go back and look at that list. Read it out loud.

Do you feel like arguing with anything on that list? How could you transform that list of negative ideas into positive gems of self-love?

_____

_____

_____

_____

_____

_____

_____

_____

_____

_____

_____

_____

_____

_____

_____

_____

_____

_____

_____

_____

_____

_____

_____

_____

_____

_____

_____

_____

_____

_____

_____

Name one positive thing about your body. Think about it and describe that positive feature here. *Bonus points awarded* if you can name two or three positive things about your body.

_____

_____

_____

_____

_____

_____

_____

_____

_____

_____

_____

_____

_____

_____

_____

_____

_____

_____

_____

_____

_____

_____

_____

_____

_____

_____

_____

_____

7. Drink Your Water from a Waterford Crystal.

Remember, treating yourself like a precious object will make you strong.

~ Julia Cameron

Eating is one of the greatest pleasures of life. Tasting exquisite food brings tremendous sensory satisfaction, and yet meals, on many days, are squeezed in around other things. We eat in the car. We eat standing in front of the refrigerator. We eat over the sink. We eat standing over the newspaper in the break room at work. Because we eat while doing other things, perhaps we become preoccupied. And that preoccupation could lead to our becoming unaware of what it is we're putting in our mouth. If we're preoccupied as we eat, after the first bite or two, food may become tasteless, and we continue eating out of habit or simply because the food is there, not because we're tasting it or enjoying it or even noticing it.

In reality, we eat not only with our mouths, lips, teeth, and tongue, but with our entire senses. We smell the aroma, we see the beauty of the food on the plate, we hear the crackling of the food cooking on the stove or in the oven, or the crunching of food as we chew it, and we feel the smooth or creamy or crispy or chewy texture of the food in our mouths. Eating can be a sensual experience, and when we feed all of our senses with beauty and pleasure, two bites of something exquisite can be more satisfying than an entire bag of Halloween candy. Sometimes I think that's why we go to restaurants. Everything looks so good! So beautifully prepared and presented!

The act of sensual eating is integral to losing weight with pleasure. Here are some ways to infuse pleasure into your meals: use your good china. Use your crystal. Use your silver. Enjoy everything about the experience. Eat with all of your senses. Consciously focus on the smell, the sounds of the food as it's cooking, the sounds of the food as you're crunching on it, or the sound as you cut into it, or the texture of it in your mouth, or the taste—engage all of your senses in your meals.

Make each bite you take an exquisite sensual experience.

Regena Thomashauer writes, "When you eat, make sure it is exactly what you wish and that you draw it toward you in the grand style, fit for a queen. If it is a potato chip, have it on your favorite piece of china. If it is cottage cheese, eat it out of your crystal bowl. You get the idea—no stuff-and-shove. Only giving yourself the full richness of your desires on a platter will do, and relish every bite. You are the queen of your desires and your world, so act like one, especially when you are the only one there to see it. You deserve the best. Accept nothing less."

Playtime: Crystal and China.

Commit to yourself that you will create a beautiful eating environment.

We each have a different perception of beauty. Some may be fine with a plastic ketchup bottle at the table as long as it's tidy and clean. Others may desire that any condiment be housed in a crystal bowl. The point is—decide what you would like to have in your environment—what kind of ambiance would bring you the most pleasure? Candles, a new tablecloth, family heirloom serving dishes or flea market finds? A technology-free zone? Quiet music? Loud music? Close your eyes and see the changes you will make to your eating environment. Write out what you imagine, and then write out your plan to create it:

8. Write A Letter to Your Fat.

One act of thanksgiving when things go wrong is worth a thousand when things go well.

~ John of the Cross

Here is a question that may feel strange. But your answer will provide you with some powerful and revealing insights.

The question: "How has your excess weight served you?"

Another way of asking it: "How has excess weight helped you?"

And further: "What benefit do you receive from carrying with you extra weight?"

"It's done nothing for me, Kristin," you might say. "My weight has only hurt me. It's only given me suffering and pain. Look at my life. My health is horrible. I haven't had sex in years. I can feel people looking down on me in my job, in restaurants, on the subway, and at the grocery store. But you want to know what's worse than all that? I'll tell you what's worse! What's worse is that I look down on myself."

On one level, I might agree with you. All of these statements may be true. You may indeed believe that your weight has given you no happiness or benefit or reward. And you may, in fact, be looking down on yourself.

However, think again. And think a little more deeply. Your extra weight probably has, believe it or not, benefited you in some way.

In fact, your extra weight may have served you very well. Perhaps your weight has protected you. Perhaps it has shielded you. Perhaps it has kept you safe.

Most people don't give their extra pounds any positive attention at all, but truthfully, those extra pounds may clearly and substantially be benefiting you! You are being rewarded by being overweight. You are, in fact, receiving a payoff. You're certainly reaping the benefit of carrying around that extra weight. And your task is to determine what that benefit is.

But here's the crux. When you allow yourself to recognize how the weight has served you, and what subconscious needs that extra weight has met, you may then move in the direction of finding other ways to meet those needs and reap those benefits.

Here's one way to figure out what those benefits might be.

Write a letter to your fat.

Here's mine:

Dear Fat:

You have been with me for so long that I thought you were a part of my destiny. Our connection has been so deep, intense, and long-lasting, that for years, I have felt you to be a part of my soul. And I thank you for the deep connection we've shared, because over the years, you have taught me very well. You have protected me with a comfortable cushion of insulation. And this insulation has kept me safe from the rest of the world.

You were also a test. You were an instant, ready-made test that I made my friends and my lovers take. If the people in my life liked me with your playing such a prominent role in my life, then I could be sure that they liked me for me. I knew they liked me for who I was on the inside, and not for what I looked like on the outside. And so, dear fat, you were a test that all of my friends successfully passed.

You were my lifestyle. Being with you felt so easy, and you came so easily into my life. I didn't have to work at maintaining our relationship. You took no effort to integrate into my lifestyle. You certainly took no energy and not much planning. You allowed me to eat anything I wanted, at any time, in any quantity. You allowed me to not plan any meals, to not control or even pay attention to what I was eating. You made it easy for me to eat whatever happened to show up in front of me. You made it easy for me to put the responsibility for my food intake in someone else's hands. And with you surrounding me, I didn't have to think of anything. I could just comfort myself in mindless eating.

You were always there for me. You were consistent. And I could count on you.

And, dear fat, you were also a way for me to fit in with the crowd. Both of my grandmothers were fat. My mother was fat. My boyfriend was fat. Most of my friends were fat. So, allowing you to be a part of my life was a way for me to be accepted by my family and friends and fit in and not draw attention to myself. You made my life easy, easy, easy!

But while we were together, it wasn't all fun and games. In addition to providing me with insulation, protection, comfort, and ease, you also magnified my feelings of depression, worthlessness, helplessness, hopelessness, and self-loathing. The worse I felt, the larger a role you played in my life.

However, just because you are a part of my life right now doesn't mean that you will always be a part of my life. I have huge desires for my body and my spirit, and I'm afraid you and I no longer have a future together. You are not a part of my desires. I can share my life with you no longer.

I do thank you for your protection, comfort, and easiness, but now it is time for us to part ways. I will always remain grateful to you for the lessons you have taught me, but we will no longer be intimately involved.

I look forward to a future without you.

Gratefully,

Kristin

Playtime: Write That Letter to Your Fat.

Now it's your turn. Write a letter to your fat. What will you say? *Extra credit*: If your fat were to write back to you, how would it respond?

_____

_____

_____

_____

_____

_____

_____

_____

_____

_____

_____

_____

_____

_____

_____

_____

_____
_____
_____
_____
_____
_____
_____
_____
_____
_____
_____
_____
_____
_____
_____
_____
_____
_____
_____
_____
_____
_____
_____
_____
_____
_____
_____
_____
_____
_____
_____
_____

9. Have a Pleasure Plan for the Bad Days.

Make a moment that is normally not fun into fun for you.
~ Regena Thomashauer

Now that you're excited about exploring pleasure, now that you're motivated to treat yourself well regardless of your current size or weight, now that you're focusing on *what will bring you the most pleasure*, now that your enthused and pumped up and excited and thrilled at the idea of falling in love with yourself and your body, now that you think that the best days of your life are in front of you, now that you really believe that you are "all that and more," you can conquer the world with your own fine, fabulous self.

But what's going to happen when the inevitable happens, when you've had a bad day?

What will be your plan?

What will be your strategy?

We all have stress, frustration, and boredom in our lives. Sometimes those bad days make us want to give up completely, throw in the towel, and say "What's the use?" Rather than abandoning ship and taking a life boat to the nearest Long John Silvers, you need a pleasure plan for the bad days.

Know that you will have exquisite days.

And know that some days will be less than exquisite.

And so, have your pleasure plan ready to go for those "less-than-pleasurable" days.

Maybe your less-than-pleasurable moment is 6 p.m. on Friday. Tired and stressed, you encounter three accidents during rush hour traffic on your way home. Your work week has been long and difficult. You hit every red light and road construction zone you could imagine. In a past, less-pleasure-centric life, your default pleasure plan would be to open up the freezer and pull out a carton of Ben and Jerry's. And while Cherry Garcia may give you a glimpse of momentary pleasure while it is in your mouth, will eating the entire container be the route to take that will give you the most pleasure? What would give you the most pleasure? Taking a walk? Having a handful of pretzels? Crunching an apple?

In my experience, there are two kinds of hunger. There's true physical hunger, where you haven't eaten in a few hours and you're just plain hungry. When one feels physical hunger, one may also experience physical symptoms, like a little emptiness in your stomach, or a growly belly, or a little nausea, or you feel a little headache coming on. Those may be messages from your body asking to be fed.

But there's another type of hunger, too. I call it emotional hunger. Emotional hunger is when you feel a certain feeling, like anger, stress, anxiety, joy, happiness, boredom—you name it—and you use food to deal with that feeling, whether it's to numb out, or relieve stress, or burn a little extra energy. You experience an emotion and then you eat to deal with that emotion. The thing about eating to deal with emotional hunger is that the eating part of the deal NEVER helps. Food will never fill you up emotionally. If there's an emotional component to your food intake, food will never truly satisfy you. If you're eating because you're sad, or upset, or stressed, or angry, you may still be sad, upset, stressed, and angry when you've polished off that plate of fried chicken. And you'll be unpleasantly full, to boot.

The Importance of Establishing a Plan for Difficult Days:

Plan your pleasure.

Allow your true pleasure to align you with your true desires.

Turn a "risk-prone situation" into a "pleasure-prone situation!"

Is the momentary stress release of eating a bag of Doritos really going to get you what you truly want? Probably not. The crunch of a chip can only get you so far and the pleasure will disappear as soon as you swallow. Ben and Jerry may not be your most worthy companions as you discover and uncover your deepest fabulousness. But planning your pleasure will.

A few years ago, I had a mammogram. I was not happy to be having a mammogram. I didn't want to have a mammogram. I put off having a mammogram.

But I ended up having a mammogram, nonetheless.

After the mammogram was done, the radiologist wanted to do a second mammogram. I did not want this either. I was not happy to be having a second mammogram. In fact, I was so obstinate about this second mammogram that I blew off returning the physician's phone call to actually schedule it.

But I had the second mammogram, nonetheless.

After the second mammogram, the radiologist wanted to do an ultrasound. That was something that I really, really, really did not want to do. At all. I was completely uninterested. I was completely resistant. Nope, didn't want an ultrasound.

But I had the ultrasound, nonetheless.

As I sat in a waiting room, shivering in an ugly hospital gown, waiting for the technician to come in and do the ultrasound, I got scared. Really, really scared. My mind started going crazy with the possible outcomes of this ultrasound. I was mentally freaking out, and all I was doing was just sitting there. I was creating, in my brain, one catastrophe after another, after another. And I started crying. Silently. It wasn't a great situation. In my mind, I had given myself Stage IV invasive cancer and was on my death bed.

I had to get ahold of myself. I didn't want to embarrass myself by looking like a blubbering fool when the technician showed up. So, in that moment, I reached for the tool of pleasure.

Where is the pleasure in this? I asked myself.

Immediately I glanced at the wall. On the wall was a photograph of a peaceful mountain scene, complete with trees, water, sky, beauty. And for the next few minutes (or however long it was) I focused on the beauty of that scene. I dove into the water, I felt the alpine air, I smelled the wild flowers, I heard the birds chirping, and created as much pleasure for myself as I could.

Eventually, the technician came in, and we got the procedure done. But for those few minutes of mental freak-out while I was waiting, pleasure was my strategy, and pleasure was my path through my mental anguish. (Ultimately, the ultrasound led to a biopsy. The tissue was benign.)

As we move toward our true and deepest desires for our bodies, know that there will be bad days. There will be awful days. There will difficult times. They will happen. It's part of being human. But having a pleasure plan for those really difficult times can be an effective strategy for dealing with life when life turns to shit.

Here are a few things that might help you in developing a pleasure plan for when the going gets tough. . .

TEN TIPS FOR WHEN THE GOING GETS ROUGH:

1. **Have a list**. I was 26 when my dad died unexpectedly. I entered therapy. My therapist said, "Make a list of things that make you happy." That was one of the best pieces of advice I've ever received.

2. **Have a pleasure plan for bad days.** I have yet to meet a person who is free from suffering. I have yet to meet a person who has never had a bad day. I have yet to meet someone who leads an idyllic life. We all have days when the unexpected happens. We all have days when challenges arise. Expect challenges, and have a strategy (or pleasure plan) for dealing with them.

3. **Treat yourself gently.** Sometimes we're harder on ourselves than anyone else is. Sometimes the most ruthless voice we hear is the one inside our own heads. When your inner critic voices her opinion, silence her with gentleness—and a bubble bath. Treat yourself kindly. Treat yourself compassionately. Treat yourself with respect.

4. **Look at how far you've come**. Consider everything you've achieved in your life. Think about what it took to make those things happen. Acknowledge the skills and tools and talents it took to accomplish what you've accomplished. Be proud of what you've done.

5. **Enjoy food.** This does not mean to eat mindlessly. This means to eat what will bring you the most pleasure in a way that will bring you the most pleasure.

6. **Touch something soft.** This could be a feather, or the fur of your pet, or a piece of velvet. Enjoy the pleasure that your sense of touch can give you.

7. **Listen to something beautiful**. Never underestimate the power of sound to transform your mood and shift your perspective, whether it's birds, Bowie, Britney, or Bach.

8. **Sniff your favorite scent.** And this doesn't necessarily have to come from a perfume bottle. Maybe it comes from lilac bushes, or a scented candle, or onions and garlic, or. . .

9. **Observe the beauty that is around you.** It is always there. Sometimes we just have to search.

10. **Be grateful.** I remember Oprah Winfrey, years ago, speaking of her gratitude journals. I thought at the time, "Yeah, that sounds fine I suppose, but I've got other things to do! I've gotta finish my dissertation and clear the cat boxes. I'll get around to gratitude later." Then after a decade or more, I got around to gratitude. What I learned? Contemplating—and being grateful for—the good in my life is one of the most effective ways to handle a so-called bad day. When the going gets tough, get grateful.

Playtime: Develop a Pleasure Plan for Bad Days

When it comes to food and eating, when do you feel the most vulnerable? Note the emotions and feelings you have when you're tired, stressed, angry, out of sorts. What sort of pleasurable plan can you have to deal with the bad days? How can you incorporate pleasure into a bad situation?

_____

_____

_____

_____

_____

_____

_____

_____

_____

_____

_____

10. Don't Hate Your Body. Love It!

You cannot love others without loving yourself.

Where do I go to learn to love myself? If I want to learn to drive a car, I take a driver's education class. If I want to learn to play an instrument, I take music lessons. If I want to learn to cook Thai food, I talk with somebody from Thailand, or I read a book, or take a class. But where do I go to learn to love myself? Where do I go to learn to love my body?

My mother didn't teach me how to love my body. Nor did I learn how to cherish myself from the media, or my teachers in school, or my friends, or my romantic partners. No one taught me how to respect my body, worship at my own temple, or treat my body as a divine vessel of infinite spirit—probably because the prevailing thought is that if we "worship at our own temple," we will become vain, narcissistic, and self-centered, and egotistical. Not very appealing thoughts.

How many negative thoughts do we have about our body each day? Probably lots. Lots and lots and lots. It is not easy to approve of our bodies. It's not easy to find the beautiful in our bodies when we're encouraged to think of ourselves as anything but beautiful.

When I was in the locker room at my gym recently, I saw a group of little girls, around the age of 8 or 9, all crowded around a mirror, criticizing their stomachs or bottoms or thighs. The problem starts very early. Of course, these children hear it from the older women in their lives. And while it was poignant to hear little, pre-adolescent girls chastise their bodies in front of each other, it is even more gut-wrenching to know that each one of them probably learned it from a mother, an aunt, or an older sister.

What are the features of our bodies we don't like? Our breasts, butts, bellies, thighs, legs, hair, skin, circles, pores, wrinkles, freckles, flesh, skin, hands. We're too large, too small, too droopy, too saggy, too poochy, too much cellulite, our butts are too big, too small, not shapely enough, and our thighs are too big—thunder thighs—legs too skinny—you can compile your own list.

Negative self-talk is destructive and sabotaging and completely undermines the quest for a pleasure-filled life. But the good thing is that if it comes from you, if you're saying these things to yourself, then it is possible for you to say different things to yourself.

It is possible for you to change things. The problem is that many of these ideas appear to be filled with the truth. And that's the problem. These negative statements about ourselves are not the truth. They're lies. And we're telling ourselves lie after lie after lie and we're believing them and making them true.

So, the quest in a pleasure-filled life is to replace the lies with truth. Whatsoever things are good, true, beautiful—think on these things. Think good thoughts about yourself. Think beautiful thoughts about yourself. Praise yourself. Take pleasure in your own company. Take delight in your own presence.

Why do we think negative thoughts about ourselves? Does it really matter why? Probably not. I heard a TV psychologist say once that "Why?" leads to "whine," and that leads to complaining, which leads to an expansion of the negative that already exists.

Perhaps a more pleasurable perspective is, "What are the thoughts I will think now?"

Our culture doesn't do a very good job of teaching us how to adore, cherish, or appreciate how precious our bodies are. No one really teaches us how to treat ourselves well. If we're women, we will probably learn how to take care of others. We will learn to nurture others. And we are reinforced by being taught how to please others and make others happy.

It is a fundamental truth that before we can love others in an emotionally healthy way, we must love ourselves. Sharon Salzburg writes in *Lovingkindness: The Revolutionary Art of Happiness,* "Love for others without the foundation of love for ourselves becomes a loss of boundaries, codependency, and a painful and fruitless search for intimacy."

Except we're not REALLY reinforced, because most of the women who sacrifice their lives and their pleasure for someone else are not getting reinforced. They're not getting what they need. They're not happy. And they hate themselves and their bodies.

How do women belittle themselves?

Women belittle and trivialize and demean themselves all the time. "I'm too old." "I'm too fat." "I'm out of shape." "I could never do that." And the sad thing about these statements is that they become self-fulfilling prophecies. How we talk to ourselves is critical in releasing weight through pleasure.

It doesn't matter who the woman is or what the woman has done— whether they've had a thriving career in corporate America or raised their children to adulthood, women tend to depreciate and diminish their accomplishments. And as we depreciate our accomplishments, we diminish ourselves.

Instead, wouldn't it be wonderful if women were taught how to celebrate their accomplishments and to celebrate themselves, to speak of their accomplishments with pride and acknowledgement and approval: "I did raise four children to adulthood! I'm a spectacular woman!" or whatever the accomplishment is.

When we make the decision to celebrate every aspect of our bodies, our lives will change.

Playtime: The Great Accomplishment List.

What have you accomplished in your life? List it all. High school graduation? Write it down. Giving birth? Write it down. Asking for and getting a great promotion at work? Write it down. Renovating a house, painting a room? Write it down. If you've accomplished it, write it down!

_____

_____

_____

_____

_____

_____

_____

_____

_____

_____

_____

_____

_____

_____

_____

_____

_____

_____

_____

_____

_____

What skills did you call on to accomplish those things?

_____
_____
_____
_____
_____
_____
_____
_____
_____
_____
_____
_____
_____
_____
_____
_____
_____
_____
_____
_____
_____
_____
_____
_____
_____
_____
_____
_____
_____
_____

Can your skills and abilities be connected to releasing weight? How?

_____

_____

_____

_____

_____

_____

_____

_____

_____

_____

_____

_____

_____

_____

_____

_____

_____

_____

_____

_____

_____

_____

_____

_____

_____

_____

_____

_____

_____

_____

_____

_____

11. What I Want Is Not in the Refrigerator.

To be happy, drop the words "if only" and substitute instead the words "next time."

~ *Smiley Blanton*

Food is food. Nothing more and nothing less. It's just fuel. Energy.

The problem is that we make it more than it is.

We give it more meaning and power than it deserves.

Food cannot really give us comfort. People, friends, relationships, animals, and cozy blankets can give us comfort.

Food doesn't really relieve stress. But freewriting (sitting down and putting pen to paper for a specific amount of time, with no attachment to what you write—just writing to see what comes out), going for a walk, or dancing naked in your bedroom can!

Food is not love. It cannot show us love. It cannot love us back. The issue is, however, that food can become very powerful when we give it more power than it deserves—when we attempt to fill deep emotional needs that food will never be able to fill, because, simply put, food is food. Food is not love.

One day, I had a particularly difficult day at work. I had had a disconcerting encounter with someone and I was stressed. I was angry. As I drove home, I was fuming. I walked in the door and went straight to the refrigerator. All I could think about was eating. I stood in front of the refrigerator, surveying its contents. As I was examining the leftover pizza, the half-eaten chicken, the box of

Chinese takeout, I began to feel even more frustrated, because it dawned on me. What I really wanted was not going to be found in that refrigerator. What I really wanted was not pizza, chicken, or takeout. What I really wanted was an easy, peaceful, calm, stress-free solution to the work situation. And that definitely wasn't going to be found in the refrigerator.

I suddenly realized that food was simply a convenient way of dealing with negative feelings. I was using food as an anti-depressant, a medication. I was using food as a way to repress or numb or suppress negative emotions. It was a way not to feel the feelings I had. It was a way to void them, not deal with them, not acknowledge them. Food was a way to cover up my negative feelings and push them away.

But we will never feel better after using food this way. In fact, we usually will feel worse. We end up feeling angry, depressed, ashamed, guilty, and upset because we failed again. And then what do we do? We want to eat more! But eating doesn't really make those negative feelings go away. They're still there. What does help those feelings pass is not to eat, but to feel. Allow yourself to feel whatever it is you're feeling. Allow yourself to know that what you're feeling is good, valid, and appropriate. It's perfect for whatever is going on in your life right now.

Food will never, ever give you love, support, or the release of stress that you're desiring. Food will only give you physical energy. Nothing more. Nothing less.

Playtime: The Food and Feeling Chart

What follows are two different ways to chart the food you eat and how you are feeling when you're eating it. Take a look at both charts and work with the one that feels most comfortable to you.

FEELING	FOOD

Perhaps you like a more narrative approach to recording your food intake and your feelings? If so, try the following. (Grab a journal to continue charting, or you can find the journal I've developed for sale on Amazon or wherever books are sold.)

What I ate:

_____

_____

_____

How I was feeling:

_____

_____

_____

_____

_____

What I ate:

_____

_____

_____

How I was feeling:

_____

_____

_____

_____

_____

What I ate:

_____

_____

_____

How I was feeling:

_____
_____
_____
_____
_____

What I ate:

_____
_____
_____

How I was feeling:

_____
_____
_____
_____
_____

What I ate:

_____
_____
_____

How I was feeling:

_____
_____
_____
_____
_____

What are you noticing by paying attention to your emotions as you put food in your mouth? Are you thinking in terms of finding other ways to deal with your emotions and feelings other than eating?

_____

_____

_____

_____

_____

_____

_____

_____

_____

_____

_____

_____

_____

_____

_____

_____

_____

_____

_____

_____

_____

_____

_____

_____

_____

_____

_____

_____

_____

12. What Can You Do Besides Eat?

Always bear in mind that your own resolution to success is more important than any one thing.

~ Abraham Lincoln

What pleasurable things can you do besides eat? Do you have anything else going on in your life besides food? I've known people—and I've been one of those people at certain times in my life—who are obsessed with food and obsess over food. There have been meals I've had with people where we start planning lunch while we're having breakfast, or we start planning dinner while we're having lunch! I look back and think, *Couldn't we find anything else to talk about other than the next meal?*

What can you do besides eat?

Create a list. Here are some things you might include on that list: reading, walking, biking, sewing, knitting, needlepointing, scrapbooking, drawing, dancing, having sex, photography, playing games, taking a delightful bubble bath with candles and music, giving yourself a facial, meditating.

And then next time you're standing in front of the refrigerator, feeling stressed, angry, bored, tired, upset, fatigued—pull out that list, pick something on that list, and do it.

Playtime: What Can You Do Besides Eat?

What are some other things you can do besides eat? List them:

13. Put the Pleasure Back in Binging.

If you have made mistakes, even serious ones, there is always another chance for you. What we call failure is not the falling down, but the staying down.

~ Mary Pickford

"Pleasure in binging? What? There's no pleasure in binging," you might say. "It just makes me feel sad, guilty, ashamed, and sometimes dirty. And then I feel like eating even more."

You've had a hard day at work, you're tired, you're stressed, and you really want to eat. You've felt your feelings. You've looked at your list of things to do besides eat. And you still want to eat. A lot. What's a girl to do? Look to pleasure for your answer.

Eat what you want. But really, really enjoy it.

Think about it.

Anticipate it.

Relish it.

Look at it. Enjoy the color. Savor it. Eat it slowly. Enjoy the sounds it makes. And enjoy the sounds you make as you eat it. Oooo and ahhhh over it. Taste and enjoy the flavor.

And squeeze as much pleasure as you can from it.

Playtime: Peel Me a Grape, or the Art of Sensual Eating.

Let's strike a bargain here. The next time you put something in your mouth, engage every single one of your senses—your vision, your hearing, your smell, your taste, and your sense of touch. Let's say you're eating a grapefruit. Notice the color of that grapefruit. Feel the texture of its skin as you peel it. Savor the sharp, biting scent as you cut into its flesh. Hear the sound the knife makes as you cut through its skin. Taste the fresh, fruity, tart tang as it lingers on your lips and mouth. Feel the pulp dissolve in your mouth as you chew slowly, and feel the sweet juiciness of the fruit. And really notice how you feel as you swallow the first bite.

Record your observations here:

_____
_____
_____
_____
_____
_____
_____
_____
_____
_____
_____
_____
_____
_____
_____
_____
_____
_____

14. Don't Lose It! Release It!

For me, words are a form of action, capable of influencing change.
Their articulation represents a complete, lived experience.

~ Ingrid Bengis, *Combat in the Errogenous Zone*

When you lose something, what do you want to do? You want to find it.

So, when you lose weight, what do you do? You go in search of that weight you've lost.

Think for a minute about the word "lose." When we lose something, the dictionary says that means we are "unable to find" something. We have misplaced something. We are "unable to maintain, sustain or keep something" We are "deprived" of something. So, if we lose weight, what our subconscious mind might direct us to do is seek out that which we are deprived of. We look for what we've lost.

So, just a little tip here. As you're moving through your weight loss journey, lose the word "lose." Try substituting "let go of" or "release."

"I'm letting go of some weight."

"I'm releasing weight."

Doesn't that feel better? You're letting go of and releasing what you don't need any more.

Playtime: Time to Release What You Don't Need.

There's a spiritual/physical exercise that I did a few years ago. I was overwhelmed with clutter in my life after having written a dissertation and having felt compelled to save every note on every scrap of paper I had written on in graduate school. A friend of mine, who was versed in feng shui, suggested that I give away or discard nine things a day for 27 days. As I was clearing out my physical space, I repeated a little mantra:

"I release what I no longer need."

"I release what I no longer need."

What physical items in your life do you no longer need? Can you release them? And is there a little phrase that you can repeat as you let go of what no longer serves you?

To get your brain warmed up to the idea of release, pick a room in your home that you would like to be more organized. Close your eyes and image what that room could look like without any of the extra "treasures" you've accumulated. Now, write a paragraph about how it will feel when you walk into your newly organized room:

_____

_____

_____

_____

_____

_____

_____

_____

_____

_____

_____

_____

Commit to a start and finish date for the project you just visualized completing:

_____

_____

_____

_____

_____

What will be your mantra while you are working on it?

_____

_____

_____

_____

_____

_____

_____

_____

15. Sex Isn't the Only Way to Have an Orgasm.

Exercise gives you endorphins. Endorphins make you happy. Happy people just don't shoot their husbands. They just don't.
~ *Elle Woods, Legally Blonde*

Sex is a great way to have an orgasm.

But it's not the only way!

Never in my wildest dreams did I ever envision myself having a runner's high, much less trying to describe it in words. Never did I expect to experience one, much less think that it would feel like sex. But it did!

It was September. I'd been running since June and I'd been meticulously following the training schedule my running mentor had given me, gradually and consistently adding time and then miles. The schedule called for long runs on the weekend. This was all new to me. Never before had I attempted to run four miles at one time. Never before had I even envisioned the possibility of doing such a thing. But because I do what I'm told (especially when I can see that it's in my best interest, when there is a pleasurable reason), I attempted what, not six months before, was the impossible. I ran four miles. Straight. Continuously. Without stopping. And the last tenth of a mile? I sprinted.

And holy moley—as I was walking, cooling down, I got off the treadmill to get a disinfectant wipe to clean the machine and my body felt like it had just had the most amazing orgasm ever. I felt spent. Relaxed. Invigorated. Euphoric. Ecstatic. Blissed out. Every cell in my body was vibrating with intense energy. It almost felt like I had been blessed with an out-of-body experience. And I couldn't believe it. It was beyond amazing. It was something that I'd heard about, read about for years. The unattainable, mythical runner's high. But I attained it and it was real! Never did I expect that I would ever feel the way I did after engaging in the dreaded e-word (exercise). Remember, I was the chubby, uncoordinated little girl who was always the last to be picked for a team at recess. But this chubby, uncoordinated little girl was now an adult woman who could create intense, ecstatic pleasure in her own body—not with drugs, booze, prescriptions, or food—but by simply moving her body in the way that it was designed to move, at a pace that felt great!

And so, on that day in September, I became hooked. If running could make me feel euphoric, I never wanted to stop.

It's important to remember that this orgasmic high did not happen overnight. It didn't happen all at once. I didn't wake up one morning and decide, "Oh, I think I'll have a runner's high today." It was months in the making. But during those months, I was having fun and creating a great foundation for this high! Every time I worked out during those months, I was feeling proud and excited. I was feeling a huge sense of accomplishment every time I logged my miles. I was feeling so amazing as I was releasing weight and receiving the complements. I was, most definitely, preparing for the high. And when the high happened, I received it with my entire body.

Sex certainly isn't the only way to have an orgasm.

Playtime: Live an Orgasmic Life, or Infuse Pleasure into an Otherwise Bad Situation.

By "orgasmic life," I'm clearly not speaking solely of sex. Rather, I'm looking at how you can infuse pleasure, joy, fun, and delight into the ho-hum doldrums of your day. It's possible.

The next time you have something unpleasant in front of you, look for the pleasure in that moment.

Stressed out from work? How can you find pleasure?

Car trouble? How can you find pleasure?

Argument with your spouse? How can you find pleasure?

Not enough money in the bank? How can you find pleasure?

Whatever problem or situation or challenge or opportunity that is in front of you, search for pleasure. Look for it. Because it's there, waiting to be recognized.

Here's a little example of what I'm talking about. . .

As I'm finishing up the final draft of this manuscript, I'm finding myself faced with a decidedly unpleasurable situation; my mother is moving into a nursing home. It's not that I didn't see it coming. I did. For years. But the time has come. It's here. She is in a situation where she can no longer live alone. She'll be 97 years old in a few months. She's confused. She's suffering from dementia. Her apartment must be cleaned out and vacated 30 days from now.

Not a terribly pleasurable experience, for her or for me, I'm afraid.

But I have a strategy. And that strategy is to infuse pleasure into every moment of the next 30 days. How?

Gratitude is a good start.

In order to best deal with the current challenges of my family situation, I have resumed a spiritual practice I have done in the past. Over the years, I have developed a highly pleasurable morning ritual. First, before I check emails or Facebook, before I do anything at all, I make a cup of fresh-ground coffee with real cream. I light a candle and I pull out two journals. As I sip my coffee, in the first journal I write out a list of gratitudes. After I'm done with that, I spend 20 minutes or so doing something that Julia Cameron in *The Artist's Way* calls "Morning Pages." Here I write whatever comes into my brain. My goal is to fill three notebook pages. I use real paper, a real pen, and get it all out. On the page.

Over the years as I work with this ritual, I've made some powerful discoveries. On the days that I make my morning gratitude ritual a priority, those days seem to go smoothly. And on the days I'm rushed and don't have a chance to attend to this practice, my days seem to be a little more challenge.

What other things am I planning on doing to incorporate pleasure into my life during this intense time of stress and grieving and busyness?

~Baths.

~Sleeping in a cool apartment under plenty of blankets.

~Eating really, really well.

~Spending a few minutes each morning on my hair and makeup.

~Writing in my evening gratitude journal every night.

~Noticing everything in my life that I have to be grateful for.

~Reminding myself of the difficult times I've moved through in the past, and reminding myself that things do, in fact, get better.

~Reminding myself of my resilience.

~Focusing a lot on positive self-talk in the form of "I am" and "I can" statements.

~And realizing that these next 30 days are special. There will be a time in my life when I will look back on this time with joy, love, gratitude, and pleasure.

Playtime: Take a Bad Situation and Make It Fun.

What are the situations in your life right now that are unpleasant? List them here:

_____

_____

_____

_____

_____

_____

_____

_____

_____

_____

_____

_____

_____

_____

_____

_____

_____

_____

_____

_____

_____

_____

_____

_____

_____

_____

_____

_____

_____

_____

How can you infuse fun, pleasure, and delight into these challenging situations?

_____

_____

_____

_____

_____

_____

_____

_____

_____

_____

_____

_____

_____

_____

_____

_____

_____

_____

_____

_____

_____

_____

_____

_____

_____

_____

_____

_____

16. Flirt with the Shoe Salesman.

Be bold—and mighty forces will come to your aid.

~ Basil King

What?

Flirt with the shoe salesman?

Is she nuts?

I knew, as I began to fall in love with my body, that I was actually going to have to move my body. I didn't want to. I didn't like exercise. I wasn't thrilled about it. But I knew I needed to move.

Because I am my mother's daughter and am cheap, I resisted buying running shoes. I didn't want to spend the money. Instead, I began to walk in Birkenstocks. And Birkenstocks are great for casual days. But as my walks became longer, I knew I needed better shoes. And so off to Target I went. I spent $30. I wanted to believe that those shoes would serve me well. But they didn't. They just created blisters on my Achilles tendon. And then I knew what I needed to do. I knew I needed to march my cute self into the shoe store and invest a little money in some good-fitting shoes.

I didn't want to buy expensive shoes. I wanted to be cheap. I wanted to make do. But being cheap and making do certainly wasn't going to help me create a great, pleasure-filled relationship with my body, or release weight, or fall deeply in love with my amazing physical self. Being cheap just got me blisters on my feet. So one afternoon, I broke down and went into the store. And in all honesty, I was embarrassed. I had already released about 20 pounds, but I had about 20 or more pounds to go. I really didn't want to encounter a sales person. What would he or she think—an out of shape woman buying running shoes? Would he think I was ridiculous? Stupid? Kidding myself?

I honestly don't know what he thought, but I was able to joke with him about how much cooler it is to buy from a real, live person than to buy online, because you get fitted. You get attention. You get someone who is going to measure your feet, ask you about your goals, evaluate your gait or stride or pronation. And you get a great pair of shoes.

What I also got from this brief, 10-minute interaction was inspiration. There was another woman in the store who was buying shoes. I mentioned to her that I was beginning a running program, and she said, "You should take this class! It's Beginner's Luck. It's for beginning runners. I'm starting a running program and I'm taking it. You should think about it!" And so we chatted about this class, which was being sponsored by the shoe store. It was a class specifically designed for very beginning runners, like me!

What is the point of flirting with your shoe salesman? The point is pleasure. Inject pleasure into the experiences you're dreading. Take a situation you anticipate as being a drag and enjoy it. Put fun into a not-fun situation and watch the energy shift. And as you create fun where you least expect it to be, you will create a new relationship with your life and a new relationship with your body. You will fall in love with your body because you are having such a great time in it, using it to have fun with the shoe salesperson, or the mechanic, or with the checkout clerk at the grocery store.

Because I was able to joke with the shoe salesman about buying shoes online as opposed to buying them from a real person, the situation relaxed. I relaxed. I opened up. And when I relaxed and opened up, a whole new world opened up with me. But that certainly wouldn't have happened without my choosing the path that would bring me the most pleasure—the path of flirting, joking, and having fun—the path of transforming a situation I had been dreading into a situation where I could have fun!

We all have situations in our lives that aren't much fun. We all have circumstances that, on a certain level, do not bring us to heights of ecstasy. In other words, we all have a certain amount of unpleasantness that we have to deal with. For me, walking in the shoe store was totally unpleasant. But the great thing is that we also have a lot of creative control over our own lives. And when we focus that control that we actually do have over our lives like a compass pointing north, when we focus our compass on pleasure, our thoughts change, our feelings change, our perceptions change, and our circumstances and external realities change. But the change—the decision—has to first come from us.

Any decision that you have to make, regardless of the problem, will be best served when you ask yourself this question, "What will bring me the most pleasure?" And then inject pleasure, joy, laughter, fun, humor, and silliness into your situation. And don't just flirt with the shoe salesman. Flirt with yourself as you fall in love with your fantastic, stunning, and remarkable body!

Playtime: Another Pleasure Infusion.

What situations are in front of you that could use a little infusion of pleasure and joy and beauty?

How can you flirt with yourself? Make yourself laugh? Crack yourself up? Sing in the car or in the shower? Dance when no one is looking—or dance when everyone is looking? Journal your ideas here:

17. Say the Loving-Kindness Meditation for Yourself!

May everyone be happy.

Several years ago, a Buddhist friend taught me the metta-mediation "May all beings be happy. May all beings be healthy. May all beings be free from danger. May all beings live a life of ease."

As my friend explained this to me, he indicated that the practitioner says it first for himself, then for a close friend, then for an acquaintance, then for an enemy, then for the world.

The idea is to expand the energy outward. But he made the point to tell me that first and foremost, before you say the meditation for someone else, you should say it for yourself. It's almost a way for you to take spiritual responsibility for yourself. And again, we're back to the idea of filling yourself up first, so you can overflow into the lives of others. In order for one to serve others, care for others, nurture others—one must first be satisfied.

But here is the important thing. It is **fundamental** that you say it for yourself first. It is **fundamental** that you bless yourself, that you wish yourself well, that you love yourself. For when you love yourself, you're then able to project love to others. You probably know people who have low self-esteem or a low self-image or who are negative or depressed or continuously unhappy. Their unhappiness and cynicism radiates and infects everyone they come in contact with. It's impossible to feel good in their presence. Because they feel so poorly about themselves, their negative energy expands.

But you also probably know people who are so at peace, or so calm, or so happy that their happiness just infects everyone around them. Their joy and laughter and contentment can fill the room and it's a delight to be in their presence. They have what I like to call an *inner glow*. And this glow is not something that can be bought. It comes from their inner life, from their spirit, from their essence. It's an energy that moves from the inside out. Because they are so content and at peace with themselves, they can radiate these feelings to others. But in reality, it's about taking care of their own needs, attending to their own desires and pleasures first, that contributes to their glow. They take responsibility for their own happiness. They aren't waiting for someone or something outside of themselves to make them happy. They just make themselves happy and that happiness radiates to others.

Here's the bottom line: do what you need to do to make yourself happy. Take your own pleasure as something of prime importance. Your pleasure must come first.

PLAY TIME: PRIORITIZE YOUR OWN PLEASURE.

How can you prioritize yourself? How can you prioritize what makes you happy?

What tends to get in your way? What are the barriers to your own pleasure (spouse, kids, parents, job, life)? How would your life be different if your pleasure came first? What can you do to make this happen, to prioritize yourself?

What will you do to ensure that you put on your own oxygen mask before assisting others?

18. A Crash Diet Is About Crashing. . . and Burning.

I didn't want to do a crash diet.

~ Beyonce

The only diet I ever went on was in 1989. It was all about food combining. You ate certain foods, at certain times of the day, and in certain combinations. I tried it for a week. And I promptly got sick.

That's when I threw in the towel on crash diets.

"Enough," I told myself.

I knew, intuitively, that this was the wrong approach for me.

A crash diet was not sustainable.

A crash diet was not something that I could do for the long haul.

A crash diet made me crash.

And burn.

When I got sick, I thought, "Never again. I will never, ever, EVER again go on a crash diet."

Deprivation? No, thank you.

Restriction? I don't think so.

Eat this food. At this time of day. In combination with this other food. Not for me, thank you very much.

Fortunately, pleasure is a much more delightful way to guide my food choices. And the answer to the question, "What will bring you the most pleasure?" will never steer you wrong.

Just say no to a crash diet. And say yes to pleasure.

Playtime: DIETS? NO! PLEASURE? YES!

What crash diets have you been on?

_____
_____
_____
_____
_____
_____
_____
_____
_____
_____
_____
_____
_____
_____
_____
_____
_____
_____
_____
_____
_____
_____

How did they go for you?

_____

_____

_____

_____

_____

_____

_____

_____

_____

_____

_____

_____

_____

_____

_____

_____

_____

_____

_____

_____

_____

_____

_____

_____

_____

_____

_____

_____

_____

_____

_____

_____

_____

What worked? What didn't work?

19. Become A Sticker Whore.

Giving credit where credit is due is a very rewarding habit to form. Its rewards are inestimable.

~ Loretta Young

I would certainly sell myself for a sticker. Maybe I didn't get enough stickers as a child. But one of the greatest pleasures in my life is setting a goal and achieving it! I like to do things. I get a great sense of pride, joy, and accomplishment from getting something done! And so, as I was learning how to fall in love with my body, and as I was beginning to inject pleasure into something that was not pleasurable for me (exercise), I knew that I myself—no one else but me—I had to recognize and appreciate what I was accomplishing. I had to give my attention to rewarding myself for a job well done! I had to give myself stickers!

Research shows that people who are successful at releasing weight keep a food journal (log, diary, tracker, whatever you want to call it), and I knew that for me to be successful, it was important for me to keep a food diary as well. And so I did. But I knew that I had, *had*, **had** to make it fun! I had to make it pleasurable—otherwise I'd quit doing it! I decided that for each day that I kept my log, I would give myself a "You did it!" sticker, or a "Good job!" sticker, or a "Well done!" sticker. (I shied away from "Nice try," 'cause I certainly wasn't "trying." I was "doing.") And then I encircled those stickers with a tiny little "Yes!" and those became a fundamental tool in my pleasurable release of weight.

I also found ways to approve of myself and my body and to recognize all the goodness that was coming to me. I remember taking a break from work, walking to Starbucks, and wearing a beautiful, light, floral cotton dress that fit me really well and showed off my feminine curves. It had a deep scoop in the back. I loved the way I felt as I was wearing it. I felt like a million dollars. And as I was walking down the sidewalk, a woman approached me from behind, and said, "Great dress! Is it vintage?" I immediately thanked her, and informed her no, it wasn't vintage. It was the internet. But I told her that she made my day. What a wonderful complement to receive—it was like getting a sticker from a stranger!

What are some ways you can inject pleasure into the aspects of releasing weight that might not be so pleasurable for you to hold on to? How can you have fun with the piece of the weight-release puzzle you might be resisting? Do you need to become a sticker whore? Do you need to acknowledge and approve of everything you're doing right for yourself?

This is one of the most important things you can do in the weight release process—bringing joy and happiness to a situation you've been challenged by.

Find your own way to make your challenges fun!

Playtime: Celebrate Every Little Thing.

No matter how small it is, celebrate it!

No matter how insignificant you think it may be, celebrate it!

No matter what else in your life may be going on at the time, celebrate everything that moves you in the direction of your desires.

If you ate half an ice cream sundae when you would normally eat the whole thing, celebrate your brilliance!

If you only ate a few almonds when normally you might choose to eat the whole can, celebrate your wisdom!

If you took a walk around the block when you might otherwise sit on the couch and watch TV, celebrate the walk!

If you chose to eat an apple rather than a candy bar, celebrate that you made a choice that aligns you with what your body really wants!

If you sat down and really paid attention to what you were eating, celebrate that you have five senses that allow you to experience food fully!

If you noticed something that made you smile, celebrate laughter, joy, and fun!

If you are alive, celebrate your precious humanness!

Sometimes we think we have to wait for a big event to have a party. Sometimes we think we have to wait to achieve a significant milestone to celebrate. Sometimes we think we have to wait for a holiday, or birthday, or graduation, or anniversary, or promotion to celebrate our lives. But I say, "Don't wait! Celebrate now!"

What can you celebrate right now? Journal about it, *then give yourself a sticker!*

_____

_____

_____

_____

_____

_____

_____

_____

_____

_____

20. When You See the Red Light, Stop!

The secret of change is to focus all of your energy, not on fighting the old, but on building the new.

~ Dan Millman

We all know what a red light is. It's a traffic light that, when illuminated, indicates that traffic should stop.

And we probably all know what a red-light-food is. It's a food, that when you're around it, is difficult to stop eating—it's one of those foods that probably shouldn't even come in the house.

For me, one of my prime red-light-foods would be a box of chocolate covered cherries. Give me one, and I'm cool. I can handle that. Just don't give me the whole box, because if I brought it in the house, the box would be empty before the day was over. This doesn't mean that I can never have a chocolate covered cherry. It does mean that having them in my house or in my environment might create a distinctly displeasurable situation. Does this mean that I never crave a red-light-food? No. What it does mean is that when I find myself craving a red-light-food, I start a conversation with myself and ask a few questions. The first question is: what is the flavor or texture that I'm seeking? Is is salt? Is it crunch? Is it sweet? Is it gooey? Is it chocolate? Is it a thick and rich texture? And then, after I identify the flavor or texture I'm after, I look for a pleasurable alternative. Once I find that pleasurable alternative, I enjoy that food, knowing that it will give me the instant gratification of enjoying that flavor or texture now, but it will also support my desire for the most pleasure by supporting me in my weight release or weight management desires.

Then I ask myself; *what am I really hungry for*? The truth is that any food can be a red-light food when I'm having red-light feelings. It's those red-light feelings that so deserve being paid attention to. At one point in my weight loss journey, I became very aware of this. I had an unpleasant encounter with a person at work. I felt victimized and that I was taking the brunt of this person's anger. I felt angry that I wasn't being heard. And I felt really angry that this person slammed the door in a fit of temper as she left my office. I had a 30-minute commute back home, and I was just livid and fuming in the car. I couldn't believe what had happened. I couldn't believe I'd been treated this way. And so, when I walked in my apartment, in my heightened emotional state, I walked straight over to the refrigerator. Even though I was following a specific weight loss program, I still opened the refrigerator door. But while I was opening it, a light bulb went on; *I'm really angry. And I'm at the refrigerator. This should tell me something.* In that moment, I drew a clear connection between feelings of anger and feelings of wanting to eat. In that moment, it became crystal clear what I did when I was angry. I ate. And I had never connected the dot. That discovery about myself— that angry feelings evoked a strong desire to eat—that was a game changer.

So, when you see the red light—**stop**. Ask yourself a few questions. Then proceed with caution.

Playtime: Red-Light-Foods.

What are your Red-Light-Foods?

_____

_____

_____

_____

_____

_____
_____
_____
_____
_____
_____
_____
_____
_____
_____
_____
_____
_____

What is it *exactly* that you think you are craving?

_____
_____
_____
_____
_____
_____
_____
_____
_____
_____
_____
_____
_____
_____

Are there any healthful alternatives that will satisfy your craving(s) and that will also satisfy your desire for a healthy relationship with your body?

_____

_____

_____

_____

_____

_____

_____

_____

_____

_____

_____

_____

_____

_____

_____

_____

_____

_____

_____

_____

_____

_____

_____

_____

_____

_____

_____

_____

21. Repeat After Me: "I'm Pretty Darn Cute."

There's something so magnificent about you.
I have been studying myself for forty-four years. I wanna kiss myself
sometimes! Because you're going to get to love yourself.
I'm not talking about conceit.
I'm talking about a healthy respect for yourself.
And as you love yourself, you'll automatically love others.

~ Bob Proctor in The Secret

What is the best compliment you've ever received? What do you like to hear people say to you? How do you like people to treat you? How do you feel when they treat you that way?

As we fall in love with our bodies and release weight with pleasure, it's beneficial to pay attention to the words we use as we talk to ourselves. And if we're thinking about falling in love, then let's think for a moment about our ideal lover and what that ideal lover says to you. What are things that he or she says to you? What do you want him or her to say? Do you want him to tell you that you're beautiful, adorable, magnificent, spectacular, stunning, brilliant, luminous, fun, funny, silly, delightful, that he loves spending time with you, that you're valuable to her, that your worthy and important to him, that your precious, and that she loves you?

PLAYTIME: List all the things you want your ideal lover to say to you.

Now, look in the mirror and say those things to yourself.

And at the end of the exercise, pick your favorite, and write it in lipstick across the mirror. Smile at yourself when you see this on your mirror!

"Oh, Kristin," you might say, "this feels so stupid. I can't do that. This is the most ridiculous thing I've ever heard of. How can I look at myself in the mirror and say, 'I'm beautiful' when I feel anything but beautiful?" And to that I say, "That's the most important time to stand in front of the mirror and acknowledge your own beauty." Go ahead and feel stupid. But do the exercise. Why? Because it's important? The concept of positive self-talk is not the most important thing in a long list of very important things. It's the only thing.

As I was falling in love with my physical self and releasing excess weight at the same time, I started walking. And as I've mentioned previously, the walking morphed into running. And the more I ran, the more I started to really pay attention to my legs. I started noticing the changes that were occurring on an almost daily basis. I could see that my muscles were becoming more firm, more defined, more pronounced, and larger and more shapely. And I loved it! Each leg was like an hourglass. As I was sitting in the bathtub, shaving my legs, I really began to notice, pay attention to, and appreciate the transformation they were undergoing. I enjoyed looking at my muscles as they were developing and feeling how hard and firm they were. I actually purchased two pairs of shorts (after not owning any for 15 years!), and what do you know? The first day I wore those shorts, a man said to me, "Nice legs." Coincidence? I think not. I know his response to my legs was a direct result of my lavishing my stunning, fantastic, and adorable legs with stunning, fantastic adoration.

When you acknowledge your own beauty, as you are right now, when you whisper sweet nothings in your ear, you lay the foundation for a legendary love affair—with yourself. Speak kindly, gently, and lovingly to yourself. Treat yourself as a sacred lover. Relish your body.

PLAYTIME: Treat Yourself as the
Sacred Object You Are:

How can you speak kindly, gently, and lovingly to yourself?

How can you treat yourself as a sacred lover?

What do you want a lover to say to you?

Can you say those things to yourself?

Extra credit: Write those things in lipstick on your mirror!

_____

_____

_____

_____

_____

_____

_____

_____

_____

_____

_____

_____

_____

_____

_____

_____

_____

_____

_____

_____

_____
_____
_____
_____
_____
_____
_____
_____
_____
_____
_____
_____
_____
_____
_____
_____
_____
_____
_____
_____
_____
_____
_____
_____
_____
_____
_____
_____
_____

Kristin Heslop

22. Gratitude? For *This* Body?

Enjoy your body, use it every way you can. Don't be afraid of it, or what other people think of it.
It's the greatest instrument you'll ever own.

~ Baz Luhrmann, *Sunscreen*

For me, it was my breasts.

For much of my life, I have detested my breasts.

They started developing when I was in third grade. Third grade!

And then, much to my dismay, they became large. Quite large. So large, in fact, an ex-boyfriend made it clear, on more than one occasion, that he found them distasteful and disgusting. So what's a large-breasted woman to do when her boyfriend doesn't dig her breasts? The only reasonable and sensible thing; I immediately went into disapproval mode. As I already had issues with my breasts, those issues were clearly being reflected back to me by the man who happened to be in my life at the time.

Thankfully, that man is gone. And thankfully, I learned how to fall in love with my body. I began to appreciate that I had two breasts, not one, but two! I came to see that my breasts are fairly symmetrical. And my breasts garnered male attention. In the past, my thoughts would have disapproved, judged, and not been in agreement with whatever male attention was focused on my breasts, because I would have found it embarrassing, disconcerting, and a turn off. "Come on, dude! Look me in the eye. Please!" But now, I realize that a man's attention to my breasts is simply a tribute to my spectacular female beauty—and my spectacular set of cans! And when it happens, I appreciate it. But here is the good news—I don't have to wait for a man to appreciate my breasts! *I can appreciate them all on my own!*

I appreciate that I have two breasts and that they're beautiful! I like their color—their pale, creamy-white color, and I like the beautiful nipples, so malleable and flexible and adaptable and supple. Sometimes they're firm, hard, and erect. And sometimes they're more soft and more spongy. I love the size of my breasts—how they look in comparison to the rest of my body. And I like that they are what really makes my body look like a woman! I like what they do for me sensually; that they are so responsive to certain types of touch that they can just almost send me out of my body. Merely by caressing them and touching them in a certain way, they can bring me to exquisitely pleasurable heights.

Women need to change their inner voices to shut down negative self-talk. What follows is an exercise designed to show you how to do that on what many of us believe is a tough topic—cellulite!

HOW TO CELEBRATE CELLULITE

As we learn to love our bodies, we learn to embrace and accept and be grateful for every aspect of our physical presence—even the ones who really don't like! So, here are a few reasons to celebrate and be grateful for cellulite.

- Cellulite is truth. It exists, whether you like it or not.

- Cellulite gives us information. It gives us great feedback about what we've been eating and how much we've been moving.

- Cellulite is objective. It doesn't judge us. It doesn't complain. It simply is what it is. Nothing more, nothing less.

- Cellulite is an efficient manifestation of body fat. Body fat is stored energy. And that's a good thing, because it means that if need be, we could survive a famine.

- Cellulite is a great teacher. It gives us the amazing opportunity to learn to embrace all of ourselves. If we can accept even parts of our bodies that are not traditionally considered beautiful, then we can move in the direction of complete and total self-acceptance. And the more we can love and respect our bodies, the more we can allow that love and respect to inform our choices about food and activity.

- Cellulite is a reminder of our mortality. According to some research), a correlation exists between between aging and cellulite. And as we are reminded that we, in fact, will not live forever, we can take pleasure and appreciate and be grateful for the life we have right now.

- Cellulite cushions and protects our bodies. Who doesn't appreciate the comfort of a cushion?

- Cellulite gives us shape and enhances our luscious, feminine curves.

- Cellulite (and body fat) helps regulate our body's temperature.

- Cellulite gives us permission to not be perfect.

Maybe there is a part of your body that you hate, that you despise, and that you are not in agreement with. How can you learn to love this part of yourself that you have detested for much of your life?

Here are some suggestions. . .

First, write a letter of gratitude to that part of your body. Maybe it's your belly. Write a thank you note to your belly! Thank your abdomen for all the ways it has served you. It has made it possible for you to live, by digesting and metabolizing food. If you have given birth, your belly is a true wonder of nature because it has nourished, created, and given life to another human being. List, appreciate, and acknowledge the many ways your belly has served you. Touch it with your hands. Touch it with a feather. Touch it with velvet and silk. Caress it. Say thank you to it. Maybe you could buy some glittery body lotion, shimmery sparkling lotion, and apply it to your belly. Enjoy the feeling of the lotion on it, feeling your skin against the skin of your belly, and enjoy the fun, sparkly, glittery beauty of it. Maybe you could buy some body jewels or little temporary tattoos, and decorate your belly with flowers, butterflies, and pretty designs, and body jewels. Go crazy! Make the designs symmetrical! Or make them random and abstract! But regardless, create a way to adore and appreciate and admire the parts of your body that you might not love right now. And see how this impacts your mood! Watch how your love of your body can set the tone and impact your whole day!

Playtime: Write a Letter of Gratitude to the Thing About Your Body that You Hate.

Now is the time to write a letter of gratitude to the thing you despise and detest and wish would go away. Is it your butt? Write a thank you note to your butt. Is it your stomach? Your skin? Your arms? Your back? Get out that pen and start writing.

_____

_____

_____

_____

_____

_____

23. How Do You Spell Success? R.E.W.A.R.D.S.

Recognize

Every

Weight release

Accomplishment—

Rewards

Develop

Success

As you move through your weight release experience, give yourself some recognition. Give yourself a little credit. Give yourself some rewards! One of my favorite ways to think of rewards is this: **Recognize Every Weight Release Accomplishment- Rewards Develop Success!**

First, what does the word *recognize* mean? The dictionary defines it with these words, "To know or be aware that something perceived has been perceived." Another way of looking at the word *recognize* could be as *acknowledge*. Acknowledge your weight release success. Give credence to it. Appreciate the amazing gift of your body, and appreciate the amazing gift you give yourself when you treat yourself well, and when you treat your physical body well. We could look at the word *recognize* in terms of validation—"to substantiate." So many times women demean themselves, their true needs, their deepest desires, and women denigrate their bodies. But when we substantiate our bodies, we give credence to the fact that they exist.

Yes. Your body does exist. And your body wants you to know that it exists. Your body wants you to substantiate it.

We can also view the word recognize in terms of "giving truth to" and giving a voice to. We can acknowledge the truth that our bodies exist, and that we're in them, and they are the foundation for our existence, and that we'd better be sure we have a damn fine foundation for the rest of our lives. And in giving voice to our bodies, we are recognizing the desires that our bodies have. Our bodies want to be healthy. They want to be cared for. They want to be well-nourished. They want to be treated with respect. They want—they're begging—they're crying out for us to love them. When we recognize and love every aspect of ourselves, when we can take pleasure in every aspect of ourselves, then we can see ourselves as being worthy of being treated well. And when we see ourselves as being treated well, we can then treat ourselves well.

The next word in this little anagram is the word *every*. The dictionary defines the word *every* like this: "Each and all single members of an aggregate; each without exception." So, in looking at your weight release experience, leave nothing out! Recognize and honor everything, no matter how large or how small. Recognize each success! Don't discriminate! Be inclusive! Have a non-discrimination policy toward your accomplishments. Recognize everything

The next idea is *weight release accomplishment.* So, what is the achievement that you're looking for? Is it a number on the scale? Is it that you took a walk today? Is it that you said, "No, thank you" when food was offered to you? Is it that you kept a written record of what you put in your mouth? Is it that you practiced portion control? Is it that you only ate foods that you liked, foods that tasted good, foods that gave you pleasure? Is it that you paid close attention to what you put in your mouth? Is it that you didn't mindless-eat, but that you really tasted and enjoyed the flavor and texture of a particular food? Is it that you paid close attention to your feelings and you didn't use food to numb them? Is it that, instead, you felt your feelings, you acknowledged your feelings, you allowed your feelings to surface and move through you, rather than trying to make them go away by eating? Is it that you paid close attention to your body and your body's feelings of hunger/hunger signals? Is it that you recognized when you were physically hungry and ate then, rather than because everyone else was eating? Is it that you passed up food? Recognize everything!

The next word to consider is the word *reward*, which is defined as "something given or received in recompense for a worthy behavior," or "to satisfy or gratify." How will you reward yourself? How will you gratify yourself? How will you treat yourself? How will you honor and pay tribute and recognize what you've done? What will you do to celebrate and not belittle what you've done? What is it that you will give yourself to recognize and acknowledge what you have done?

Our next word, *develop*, is defined as "to expand or to realize the potentialities of; bring gradually to a fuller, greater, or better state; to elaborate or enlarge." Rewards will help *enlarge* our weigh-release success. Also, I like to focus on the word "gradually" which has the connotation of an ongoing journey, a path, a road, and maybe not the ultimate destination. I also like to think of the word *develop* in terms of growth, nourishment, and expansion.

How can we develop and encourage growth, nourishment, and expansion in terms of weight release and rewarding ourselves for our accomplishment? As we nourish a baby, and the baby grows, so we must nourish our capacity to experience the pleasure of being in our bodies. How can we expand and magnify our weight release accomplishments? Put a lot of attention on them. Think about them. Make a list of everything wonderful you've done to release weight. And think of how wonderful you feel, either as you're doing the activity, or after you've done the activity. Praise yourself. Honor yourself. Pay tribute to yourself. Appreciate yourself. And say these things out loud—to yourself—in the mirror! How can you feed your accomplishments so you get more? Write yourself a letter of gratitude! Leave love notes to yourself hidden in special places. Speak to yourself positively and adoringly and lovingly and supportively.

Then finally, we have the word *success*, which is "the achievement of something desired, planned, or attempted." Is your definition of success simply weight release? Is it a number on the scale? Or is it a feeling of self-esteem? Or power? Or pride? Is it perhaps a feeling of joy, and pride, and accomplishment? Is it simply that you feel amazing? Is it liking what you see when you look in the mirror? Or is it approving of yourself? Accepting yourself? And if it is approving or accepting of yourself, then this is completely and totally where it all starts! Approving of yourself! Falling in love with your body! Loving yourself where you are right now, and when you do that, everything will fall into place.

Playtime: Rewards.

Create a system of non-food rewards to recognize every accomplishment you have on your weight-release journey. What do you want to recognize? A number on a scale? A size change? A behavior? And how can you reward yourself for moving in the direction of your desires, including your desires related to weight?

GOAL	REWARD

GOAL	REWARD

24. Commit an Act of Faith and Throw Out Your Fat Clothes.

The most important relationship in your life is with your body.

I know! I know!

It's hard.

You want to keep them. You've spent good money on them. Some of them are really nice. You're attached to them.

But when you think about it, why do you really want to keep them? Do you want "just in case" clothes? Just in case you ever need them again. Does it mean that you want to keep them around just in case you fall out of love with your body, just in case you start to slip a little bit, just in case you totter down the slippery slope and fall into the pit of self-loathing, just in case you recapture some of the weight you've released. And you do know what's going to happen, don't you? You'll end up back in these clothes. Because you prepared for it. Because you didn't realize that what helped you release the weight is what is going to help you keep the weight away from you, as you no longer need it! It no longer serves you.

It can be scary to throw out those clothes. They were such a big part of your life for such a long time, and you have become attached to them. Maybe those clothes have a sentimental value. Maybe they mean something to you. You remember wearing this dress at some significant event in your life—or whatever. But what means more to you? Your past, where you weren't really all that happy to begin with? Or your future, filled with love, joy, and pleasure, all directed at you and your beautiful body?

For me, throwing out those fat clothes was a very scary thing to do, because at that point, I had lost about 30 pounds. On the one hand, I knew if I kept them around I would slowly but surely, attract back to my body all the weight I had so pleasurably released. That certainly would have brought me no pleasure.

So as I grappled with what to do with my fat clothes, I asked myself, "What will bring me the most pleasure?" For me, what would give me the most pleasure was to purge my closets of all the fat clothes which had served me so well for so many years. It pleasured me to fold them all neatly and put them in trash bags and take them to my local Goodwill. My big desire was not to have any clothes in these large sizes in my apartment. There would be no revisiting the past. The past was not pleasurable, when I looked at it honestly. When I was at certain sizes, I was miserable on one level and I knew intuitively that it would not be in my best interest to keep those clothes around that I had worn when I was sad, depressed, and frustrated. I knew that my weight release efforts needed to be rewarded, and I chose to reward them by only having clothing that fit my current body.

You really do get what you prepare for. If you prepare for success, or pleasure, or love, that is what will show up. And so, by getting rid of your fat clothes as you fall deeply in love with your body, you will be preparing for and setting the stage for fitness, health, and fun!

Your fat clothes are an insurance policy you don't need. Wouldn't it be much more pleasurable to look at your closet, or your dresser, and know that they are filled solely with clothes that fit you now? Your old clothes are who you were—then! But you're not that person any more. That person didn't know then what you know now—that the most important relationship in your life is with your body, and that your beautiful, adored body would much prefer clothes that fit her and flatter her!

Playtime: Cancel That Insurance Policy.

Throw out your fat clothes.

Do it! Do it now!

Are you having trouble with this assignment? Here are some suggestions that may make the process more comfortable.

Identify the emotions you have attached to your clothing. Are you concerned about the money you spent on them? How could you address that concern? Selling them on E-Bay? Putting them in a consignment store? Taking a tax-deduction when donating them to a non-profit organization?

_____

_____

_____

_____

_____

_____

_____

_____

_____

_____

_____

_____

_____

_____

_____

Are there memories associated with the clothing? If so, how could you preserve those memories in another way? Could you take a photo of the item? Write about the memory? Meditate on being thankful for the past but ask for help to live in the now?

Practice gratitude for having what you needed when you needed it and reflect on how the clothes that you are releasing will bring pleasure to a woman who may not have the money to buy clothing.

_____

_____

_____

_____

_____

_____

_____

_____

_____

_____

_____

_____

_____

_____

_____

_____

_____

_____

_____

_____

_____

_____

_____

_____

_____

_____

_____

25. Staying the Course Over Rough Terrain.

Stick to the fight when you're hardest hit.
It's when things seem worst that you must not quit.

~ Edgar Guest

The journey of releasing weight is, truly, a journey with no destination. Sure, there may be a number on a scale, or a certain size, or maybe a set of measurements, or even a pair of jeans that may beckon you. But how do you maintain what it is that you've achieved once you've achieved it? The journey of maintenance can prove to be even more challenging than the journey of releasing weight.

So here are a few ideas that may help as you continue to develop a loving, long-term, committed, sustainable relationship with your body.

TIP ONE: A few chapters back, you developed a Pleasure Plan for Bad Days. Use it. Know that you're not perfect. Know that "bad" days are normal. Know that things may not always work out the way you think they should. But know that you can infuse pleasure into any situation.

For example, I knew that I had to have a Pleasure Plan for exercise. I knew that getting up and getting out and moving my body was not going to come naturally or easily. So, my Pleasure Plan included ways to make walking fun. On my walks, I decided to take great pleasure in the gorgeous neighborhoods, the trees, the flowers, the cats, the bunnies, the squirrels, the goats, the ponies, the lambs, the camels, the peacock (I live near a children's zoo), the kids, the men, and the women I encountered. Making the decision to experience pleasure before I headed out the door made me want to keep heading out the door!

TIP TWO: Continue to be committed to changing your language, because as you change your language and your words, you'll change your thinking and your life. Abandon any idea related to "willpower" and "self-discipline." Instead, focus on "commitment" and "belief." Here are a few ways I refocused certain thoughts:

"I just don't have any willpower" became "I'm committed to loving my body by moving it!"

"Where's my self-discipline?" became "I am filled with belief that I am headed in the right direction."

"I hate to exercise!" became "My body thanks me every time I move it!"

"I just can't say no to food" became "I only eat foods that I really, really like."

TIP THREE: Know that you're in this for the long haul (the rest of your life). Expect that some days will be easier than others. Enjoy and relish the easy days. And slow down and be gentle with yourself when you encounter rough terrain.

Know that developing a great relationship with your body is a life-long journey and enjoy the trip! Know that everything you've done to release the weight is what it will take to stay the course—knowing what it is that will bring you lasting pleasure. Treating yourself kindly and with love. Acknowledging your body for everything it allows you to do. Knowing what it is that you really, really, want. And knowing that sex isn't the only way to have an orgasm.

Playtime: The Ongoing Power of Desire.

What do you want? Continue playing with desires for yourself and your body. Your desires for your body, and for yourself, may change and evolve over time, and that's fine, because we as human beings change and evolve. But being aware of what we want, what outcome we're seeking, what the result is that we're going for, and keeping our eyes on the prize will only bring good things to us.

What do you really, really want?

_____

_____

_____

_____

_____

_____

_____

_____

_____

_____

_____

_____

_____

_____

_____

_____

_____

_____

_____

_____

_____

_____

Kristin Heslop

Refer to this handy reference guide when you need a quick reminder of the principles in this book.

Principle One:
Always ask yourself the most important question: "What will bring me the most pleasure?"

- This is important because it prioritizes things and gives perspective.
- Related to food, not all foods are equally pleasurable.
- Determine what you adore and eat that.
- Don't eat foods you hate or foods that are "good for you" just because they're good for you.

Principle Two
Eat only food you love.

- All chocolate is not created equal.
- This encourages you to taste and enjoy all aspects of food.
- If you don't like it, don't eat it.
- And when you don't adore it any more, stop eating it.
- Pay attention to feelings of fullness and satisfaction.
- Make every meal fit for the queen that you are.

Principle Three
Celebrate everything.

- Everything.
- No exceptions.
- If it's in your life, celebrate it.
- This means everything about your body, even the parts you don't like.

Principle Four
Be grateful for your body.

- Every day, thank your body for what it has done for you.
- Bless it.
- Love it.
- Truly appreciate it.
- Create rituals around it.
- Acknowledge how it has served you.

Principle Five
Complete the food/feeling chart every day.

- If it goes in your mouth, write it down.
- And before you write it down, figure out what you're feeling.

REFERENCES

Anand, Margo *The Art of Sexual Ecstasy: The Path of Sacred Sexuality for Western Lovers*, Jeremy P. Tarcher, 1990.

Byrne, Rhonda *The Secret,* Simon and Schuster, 2007.

Cameron, Julie *The Artist's Way*, Penguin Group, 2002.

Lanker, Brian *I Dream a World: Portraits of Black Women Who Changed America*, Henry N. Abrams, 1989 (Adapted from Oprah Winfrey: "I know that you cannot hate other people without hating yourself.").

L'Engle, Madeleine *Walking on Water, Reflections on Faith and Art*, Random House, 1972.

Maggio, Rosalie *Beacon Book of Quotations by Women*, Beacon Press, 1994.

O Magazine, January 2001, p. 22.

Roth, Geneen *When You Eat at the Refrigerator, Pull Up a Chair: 50 Ways to Feel Thin, Gorgeous, and Happy (When You Feel Anything But),* Hachette Books, 2010.

Siegel, Bernie S. *Love, Medicine, and Miracles*, Harper & Row, 1989.

Thomashauer, Regina *Mama Gena's School of Womanly Arts, Using the Power of Pleasure to Have Your Way with the World*, Simon and Schuster, 2002.

ACKNOWLEDGMENTS

Thea, thank you for your belief in this idea, your wicked editing skills, and your willingness to let me shrivel up my body in your hot tub. Charlene, you do know that your willing and listening ear, your broad perspective, and your practical wisdom play a vital role in my life. Thank you. Samantha, your flexibility and understanding and willingness to let me cry in your office when I need a good cry is so appreciated. Thank you for forcing me to go to the Orkney Islands. Summer, your skills are second to none. Thank you for letting me wail in your office on November 10, 2016. Susan, you've been there for decades, through good times and bad. I am so, so grateful for our friendship. Regena Thomashauer, you started this ball rolling for me back in the spring of 2007. I am indebted to your vision and willingness to speak the truth. And Maggie Hilt, though you are no longer with us, know that you were my favorite high school teacher. Thank you for fostering my love of words.

ABOUT THE AUTHOR

Kristin Heslop, DMA, has gained and lost over a thousand pounds throughout her life. A musician by trade and training, Dr. Heslop attended Union College in Lincoln, Nebraska. She holds a Master of Music degree from Wichita State University, and a doctorate from the University of Nebraska-Lincoln

Dr. Heslop has taught at Enterprise Academy, Wichita State University, Union College, Concordia University, and the University of Nebraska-Lincoln, and has performed on the flute, piano, harpsichord, and organ throughout the Midwest. In addition to music, she derives great pleasure from political and environmental activism, creating colorful visual art, and hearing her cat Lukas purr. She resides in Lincoln, Nebraska.

Stay in touch at www.kristinheslop.com and on
Facebook: Kristin Heslop, Author